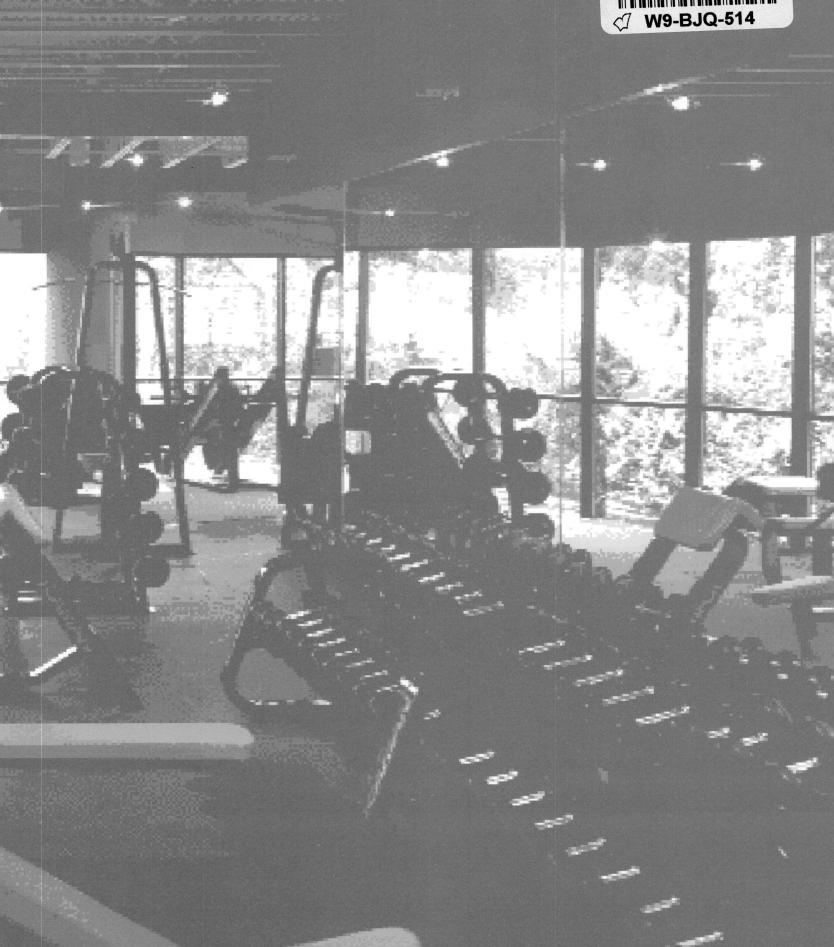

HEALTH CLUBS

architecture & design

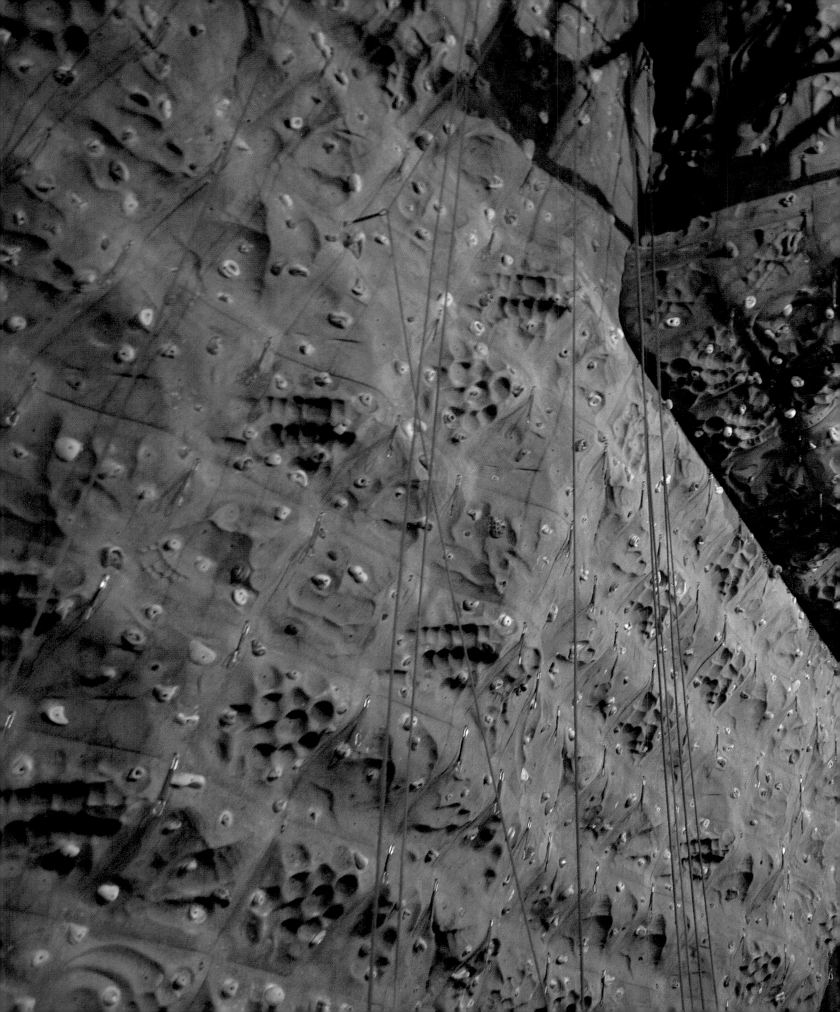

HEALTH CLUBS
architecture & design

Kate Hensler Fogarty

PBC INTERNATIONAL, INC.

*Distributor to the book trade in the United States
and Canada*
Rizzoli International Publications Inc.
through St. Martin's Press
175 Fifth Avenue
New York, NY 10010

*Distributor to the art trade in the United States
and Canada*
PBC International, Inc.
One School Street
Glen Cove, NY 11542

Distributor throughout the rest of the world
Hearst Books International
1350 Avenue of the Americas
New York, NY 10019

Library of Congress Cataloging-in-Publication Data
Fogarty, Kate Hensler
        Health clubs : architecture & design / by Kate Hensler Fogarty.
        p.   cm.
        Includes index.
        ISBN 0-86636-643-1 (hardcover). — ISBN 0-86636-644-X (pbk.)
        1. Physical fitness centers—Design and construction.
    2. Physical fitness centers—Directories.   I. Title.
    GV428.H46   1998   98-9645
    725'.85—dc21   CIP

CAVEAT—Information in this text is believed accurate, and will pose no problem for the
student or casual reader. However, the author was often constrained by information
contained in signed release forms, information that could have been in error or not
included at all. Any misinformation (or lack of information) is the result of failure in these
attestations. The author has done whatever is possible to insure accuracy.

10 9 8 7 6 5 4 3 2 1

Printed in Hong Kong

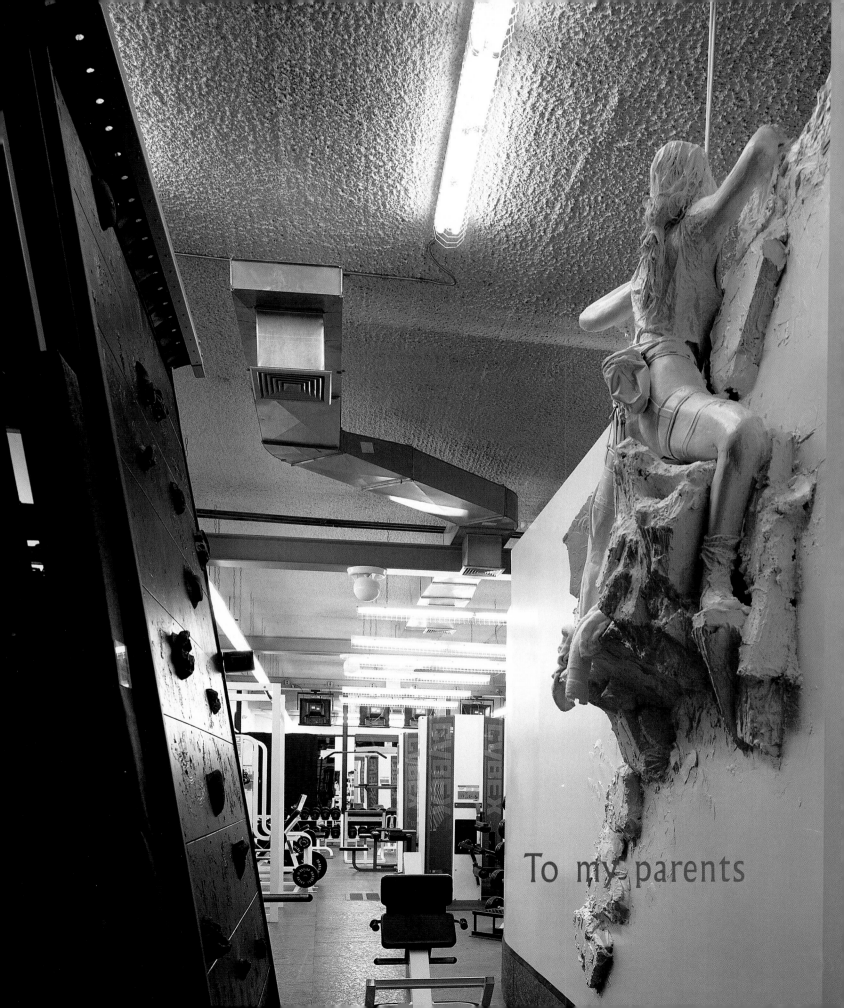

To my parents

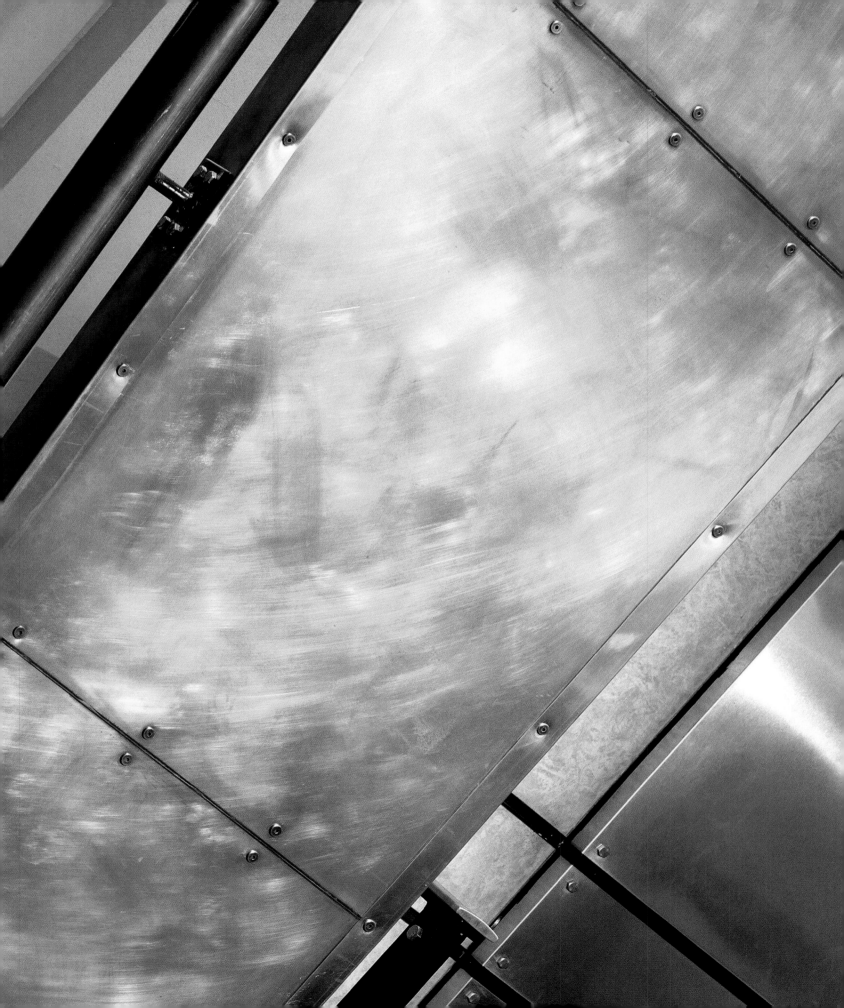

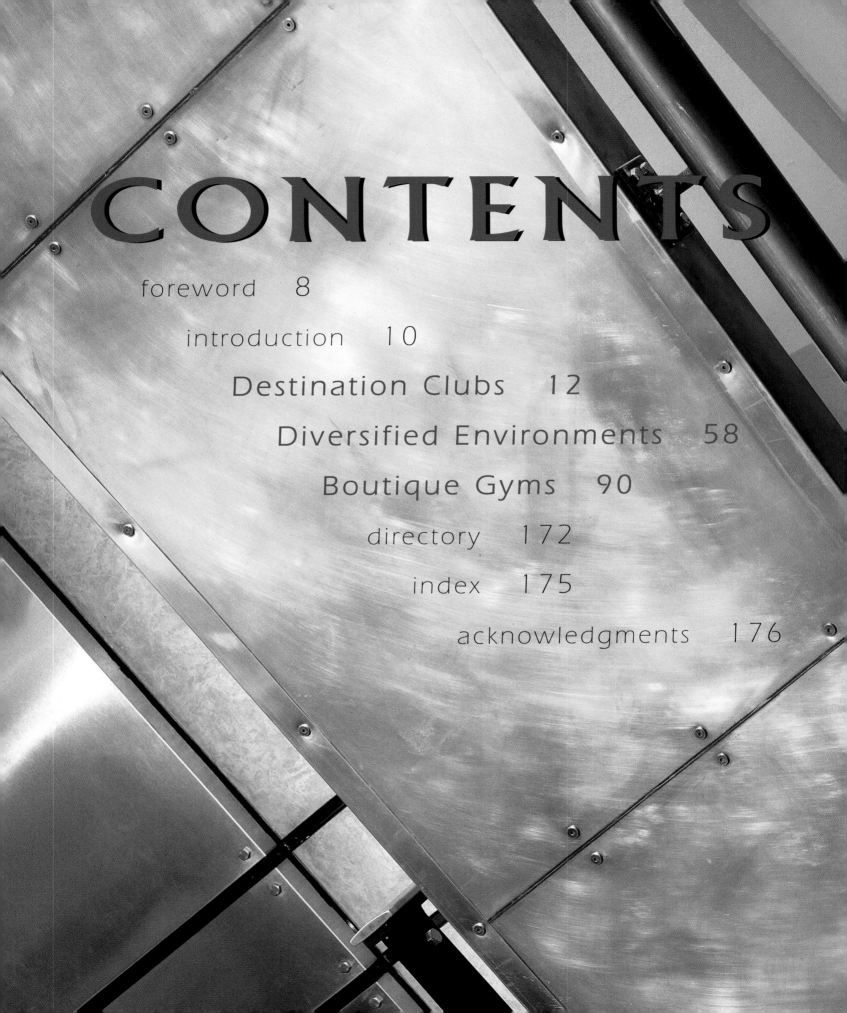

CONTENTS

An interview with
Vito Errico
co-owner / director of design
Equinox Fitness Clubs
New York City

Along with his siblings Danny and Lavinia, Vito Errico is owner of Equinox Fitness Clubs, a New York City-based health club chain that is one of the industry's most influential and successful companies. Founded in 1991, Equinox also offers its own vitamin and skin care lines, as well as three beauty spas. Vito Errico is director of design for Equinox, and has worked with some of New York's hottest designers to attain a level of aesthetics that is matched by few in the health club field.

Why is good design important to a health club?

Design is one of the three most important factors: the others are customer service and programming. The machines are the machines. It's the architecture of how they are configured that makes the difference. Clients often spend two hours a day in the gym, and they want a pleasing environment. And they have trained eyes: their homes, offices, restaurants, and stores are professionally designed, and they are attuned to architecturally pleasing spaces.

The club's design is also part of a larger identity. The packaging of our vitamin line resembles the clubs. The skin care line recalls the spa interiors. It's about the whole image, right down to the soap dispensers. Everything is graphically considered, and everything has the Equinox logo. We even scrutinize the size of the logos on our T-shirts. If you want to get to a certain level, that's what's necessary, nothing less than total design.

What is the role of the owner in a health club's design?

I bring the feeling that we want, set the tone, and work through the whole concept. The architect translates our work session into an "architecturally correct" statement.

Does good design sell memberships?

Yes. Factors like service and price are essential, but good design is like a halo that sits over the customer while they're deciding whether or not to join the club. It closes one door.

WORD

Explain the process of designing a club.

We find a space, and then start the programming process with the architect and designer. Next we allot square footage to each component and determine the flow from entrance to exit. Then comes the fun part: the details. No matter where you look there's been thought put into that space. The finishes really convey the feeling of each space and the club in general. I'm even going to design trade shows this year to research new materials. Do I get too deep into it? I do. But I think that's what sets us apart. I don't mind spending to get the look.

Discuss design of the secondary spaces.

In the locker rooms, cleanliness is the most important factor. We invest in our locker rooms. Less is more when it comes to color; everyone likes white or a shell color and it's cleaner looking. We use woods that lend a natural, luxurious touch. For the retail and restaurant components, I'll spend time in similar outlets, like Dean & DeLuca, and observe their counter service and how food is displayed and presented. These spaces are perhaps only 500 square feet of a 35,000-square-foot space, but it's often people's first introduction to the club. The architecture stays basically the same.

How do you draw the line between aesthetics and practicality?

I'd rather a club achieve 85 percent of the design vision and 100 percent efficiency. My greatest objective in designing a club is to ensure that it looks as good from day one as it does five years later. For example, a quartzite flooring we used in one club achieved the design I wanted, but it turned out to be very porous and a nightmare to clean; it's hard to use a natural stone in a club with this much use. For our newest club, I found a tile that resembles quartzite, but its efficiency is greatly improved.

What changes have you seen in health club design?

Clubs have grown in size. There are less aerobics classes, more yoga. Spas, yoga, and retail components are taking up more and more of the interior. The equipment itself only really changes every eight to ten years.

If you haven't been to your health club recently, you've probably missed its evolution from a poor substitute for a walk in the park, to a shrine to health and wellness. In this new parallel universe, accountants are boxers, doctors are marathoners, and retirees are rock climbers, reaching physical and mental goals in and beyond the gym.

These ingenious environments are some of the most exciting design projects in recent years. As the popularity of health clubs grows exponentially, so do the expectations for their aesthetics, amenities, cleanliness, and comfort. These projects make designing a living room seem like a luxury. Sofas are easy; inspiring someone to run four miles (for the fourth time in a week) or lift fifty pounds is hard.

Many designers have risen to the challenge. Health club principles like motivation, speed, intensity, voyeurism, and teamwork are explored and manifested in today's

INTROD

best examples. From coast to coast (but especially on the coasts), from the established to the ingenues, America's design firms are envisioning a new kind of club. Lighting, materials, palette, and programming are being implemented in unusual ways to answer the question: What makes people run?

The clubs reflect the society and neighborhoods they serve: The Sports Clubs in New York and California designed by J. Kent Walker Design and Langdon Wilson Architecture Planning exemplify the multi-level, multi-feature club-as-resort concept, while Thanhauser &

The faded grandeur of the former ballroom of the Hotel des Artistes in New York inspired the elegant La Palestra, designed by health club pioneers HLW International, while the Raleigh Hotel Fitness Center's tented outdoor gym mirrors the sunny, stylish rebirth of Miami's South Beach. New York's David Barton Gym, designed by Aero Studios, employs sumptuous materials and intimate spaces to create a nocturnal mood. As the club concept becomes big business, designers are increasingly required to integrate retail, dining, office, and childcare facilities as well.

Hotels are rethinking their commitment to exercise facilities, since business travelers and vacationers alike now expect clubs equal to or better than theirs at home. New, luxuriously designed spaces, crafted by some of today's best designers, can give a

UCTION

hotel new life and a new guest base. Companies of every size and sector are offering health clubs as well, their investment returned in happier, healthier employees, and a powerful new recruiting tool. Wellness centers combine principles of exercise and medicine, and have their own specific design needs, as "well" members inspire "patients" on the road to health. The clubs on these pages represent the first wave of health clubs by architects and interior designers, both in the U.S. and abroad. They are as diverse as the members they serve: small and large, opulent and pared-down, private and social. There's only one downside: With gyms like this, there's no excuse not to exercise.

—Kate Hensler Fogarty

Large health clubs or sports malls promise—and deliver—something for everyone. A diversity of services allures members of all ages and fitness levels to spend an hour or the entire day.

DESTIN

CLUBS

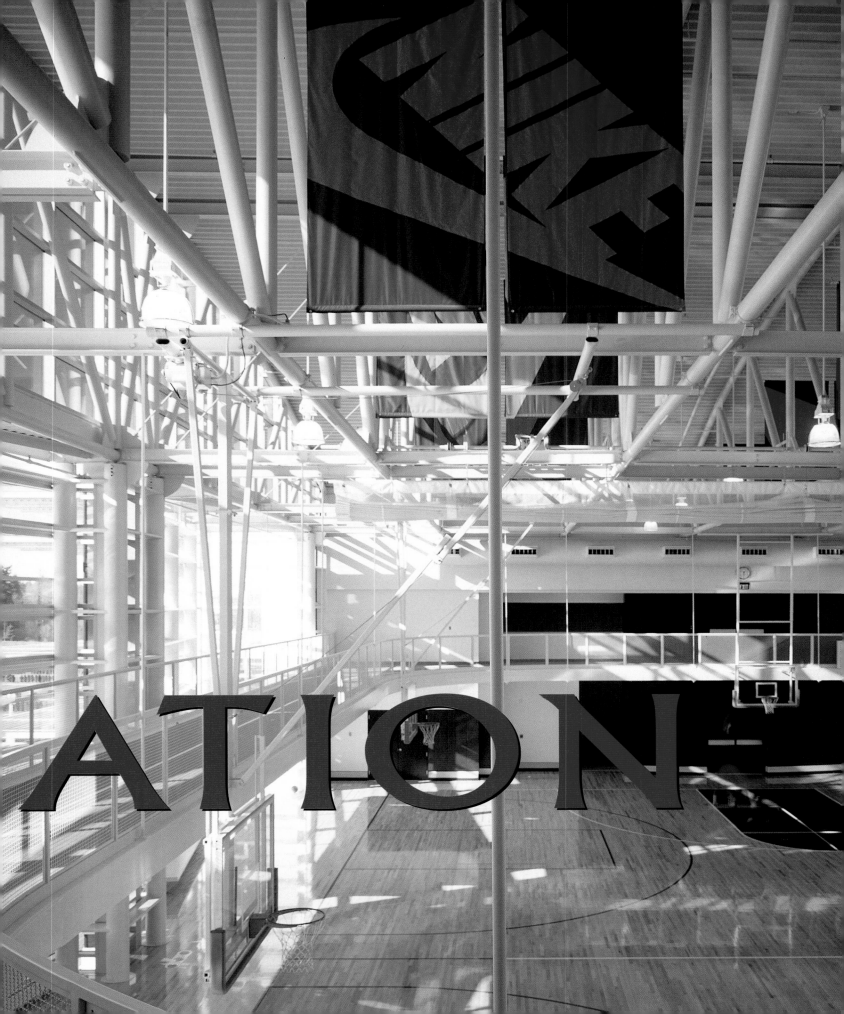

ATION

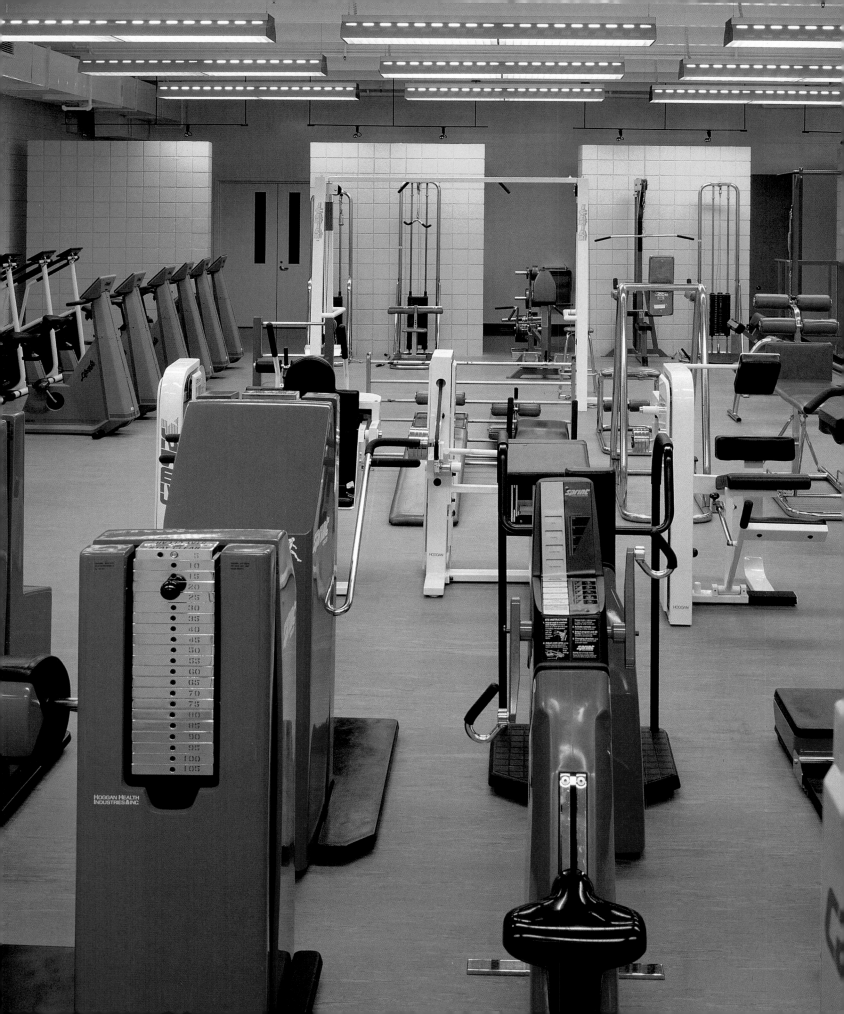

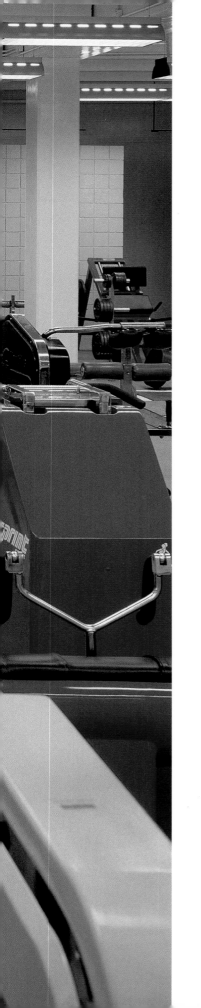

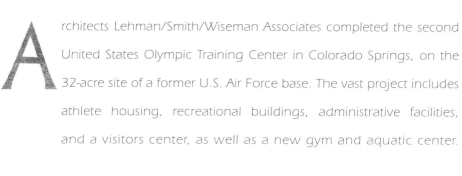

rchitects Lehman/Smith/Wiseman Associates completed the second United States Olympic Training Center in Colorado Springs, on the 32-acre site of a former U.S. Air Force base. The vast project includes athlete housing, recreational buildings, administrative facilities, and a visitors center, as well as a new gym and aquatic center.

For the gymnasium, the designers were enlisted to house the training of athletes of numerous disciplines all under one roof. Considering the complexity of the project and tight budget, the "essential functional elements were the tools available for expression," says principal W. Kenneth Wiseman. On the main level, 11 sports— badminton, basketball, boxing, fencing, gymnastics, judo, roller skating, table tennis, taekwondo, team handball, and wrestling—are

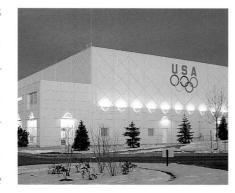

accommodated. Locker rooms, team meeting areas, video taping, video analysis, offices, and equipment storage are also on the main floor. On the lower level are three small gym rooms, one of which can be used by five sports in a multipurpose configuration: boxing, fencing, judo, taekwondo, and wrestling. The remaining space is dedicated to the weight training program. The Sports Medicine and Science Center is adjacent to the gym. The aquatic complex boasts the most technologically advanced pool in existence. Though designed primarily as a training facility, the pool also accommodates water polo and synchronized swimming, disabled athletes, and has more than 1,000 spectator seats. The complex was selected as the 1998 Foremost Sports Facility of the Year.

U.S. OLYMPIC TRAINING CENTER

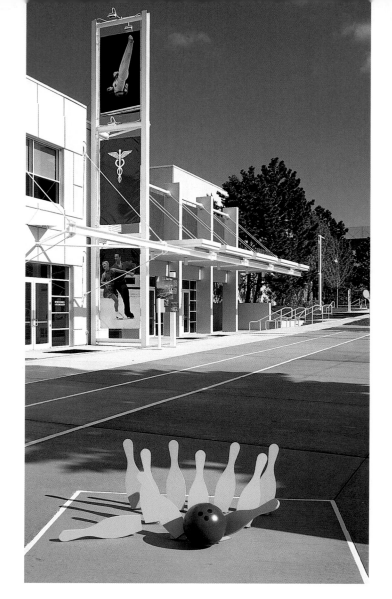

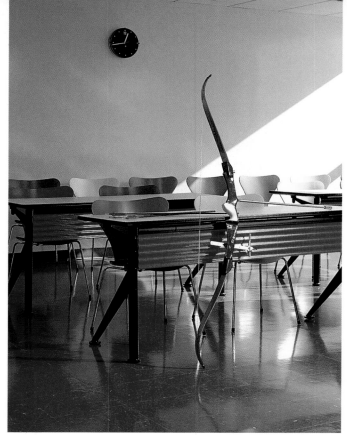

PREVIOUS SPREAD In the weight room, yellow monoliths define circulation space from the training room. Light fixtures are used as an organizational element. A sports flooring system protects athletes from shock. On the gymnasium and aquatic center, precast panel detailing organizes the facade and reduces the scale of the large volumes. ABOVE The repetitive placement of lighting and fenestration creates a strong rhythm on the building's exterior. ABOVE RIGHT A team meeting room, finished in Olympic colors, offers flexible seating and tables. RIGHT The rehabilitation area in the sports medicine center allows viewing through corridor windows; the five Olympic colors of red, yellow, green, blue, and black are visible as accents. OPPOSITE Table tennis balls are used as a wall decoration in the gym's second-floor lobby, exemplifying the use of athletic equipment throughout for decorative purposes.

location: Colorado Springs, Colorado
architect/interior designer:Lehman/Smith/Wiseman Associates, LLC
photographer: Jon Miller/Hedrich Blessing
square feet/meters: 75,000/6,968
design budget: $9.2 million

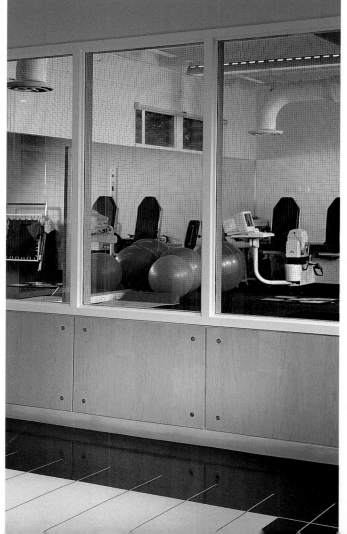

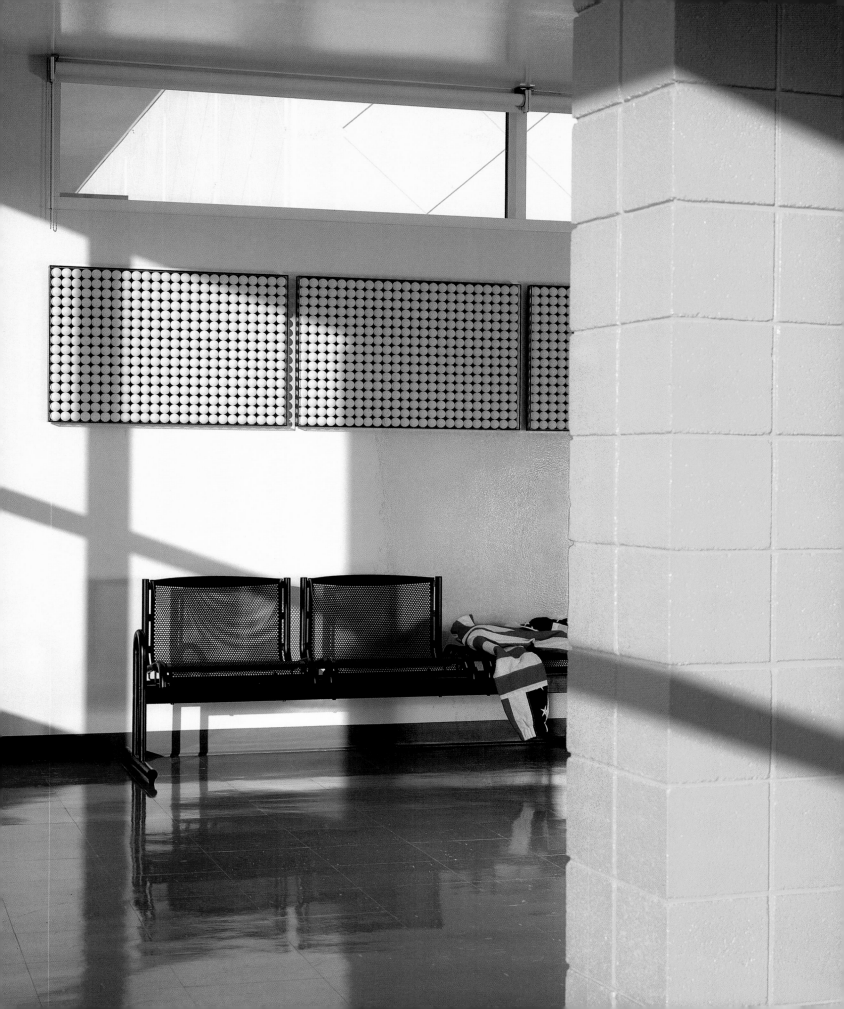

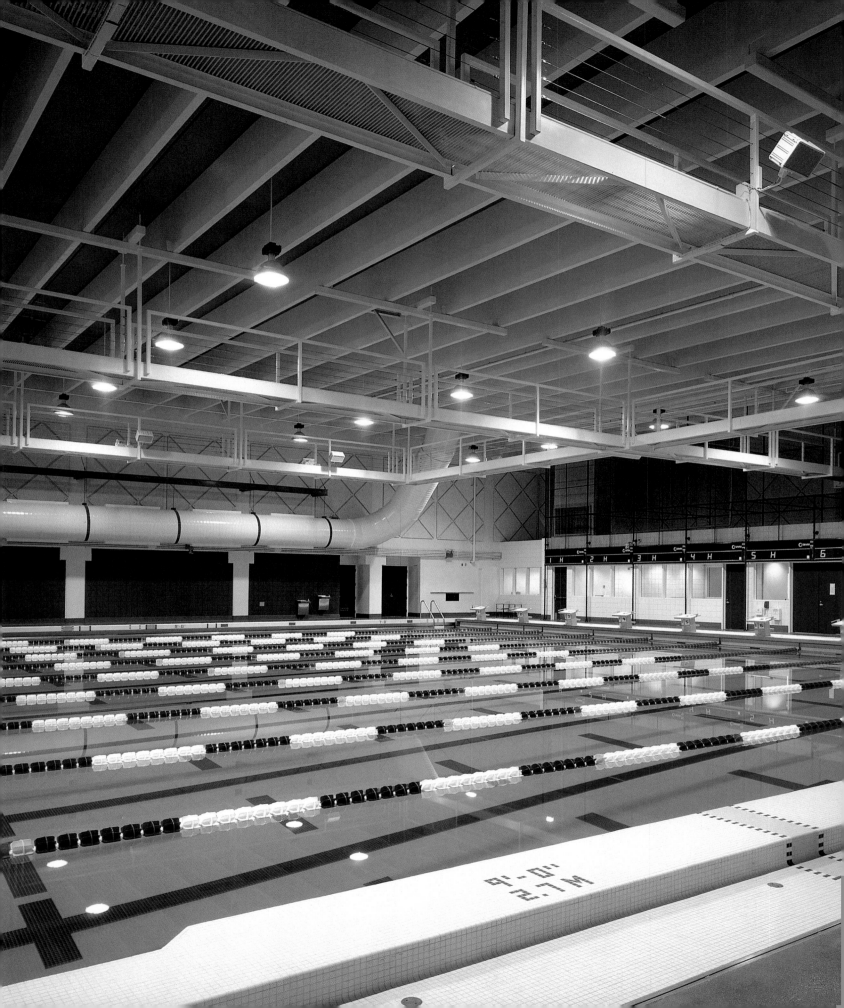

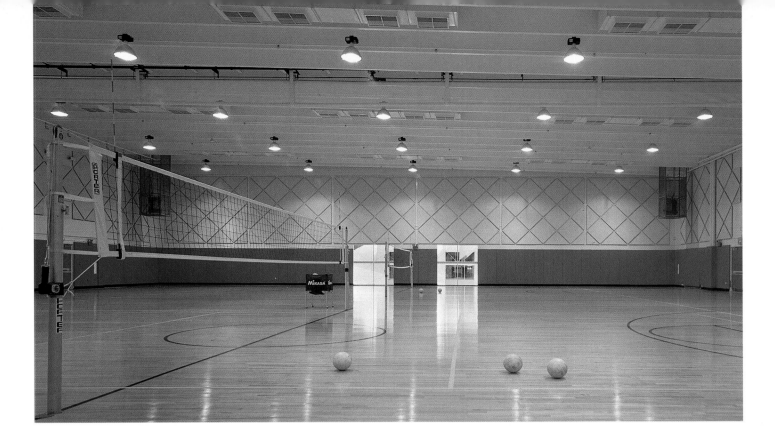

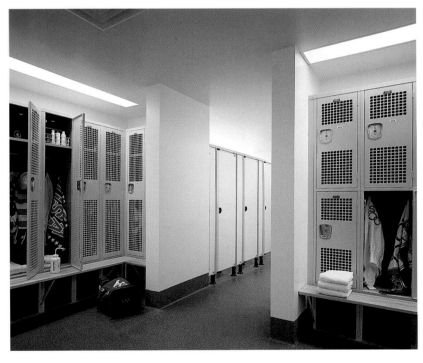

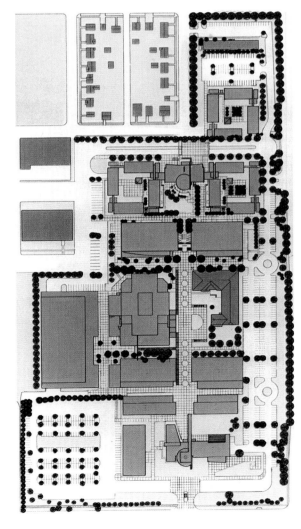

OPPOSITE The pool interior is "a marriage of a Spartan budget with many owner requirements," says Wiseman. Coaching and sports science offices compose one side of the perimeter overlooking the pool area. The video system is connected to the complex's cable TV network, which allows access for analysis in the sports science center, coaches' offices, or dormitory rooms. **ABOVE** In the gym, acoustical panels were shaped and rotated to mimic the pattern of the exterior precast. Red chain link enclosures protect equipment, while red protective mats form a base for the room. Viewing windows allow visitors to watch training activities. **ABOVE LEFT** The Olympic colors are used as accents in locker rooms and changing areas.

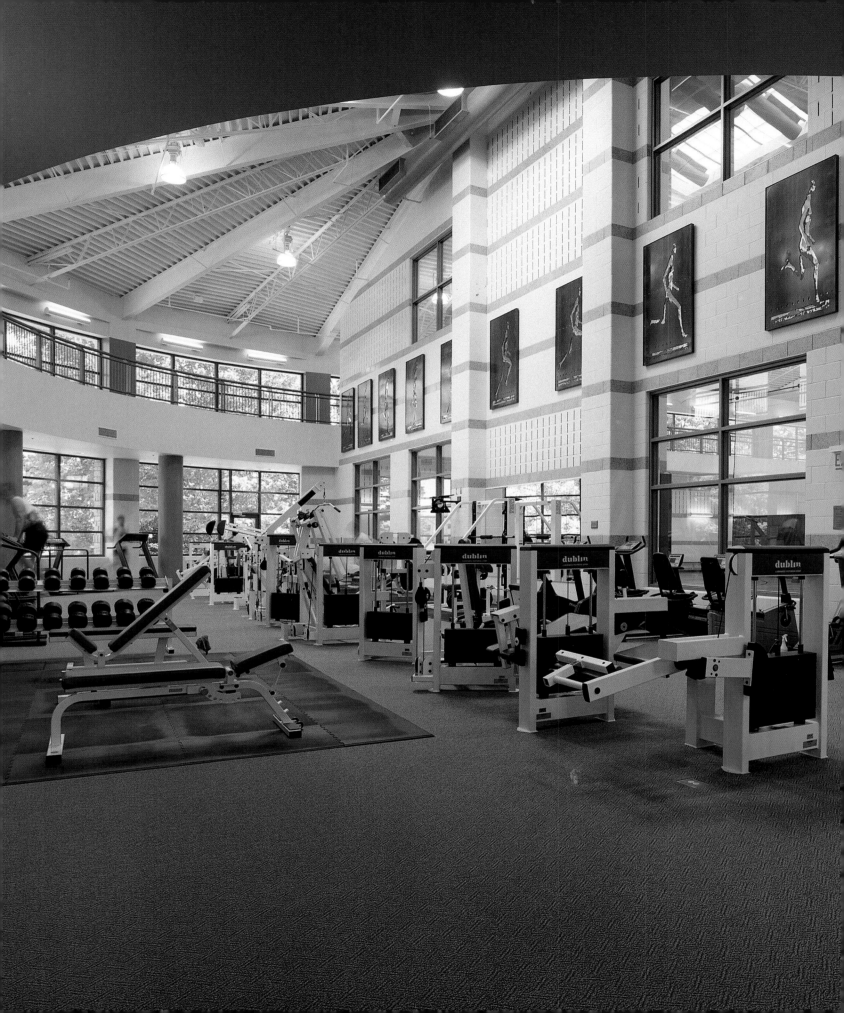

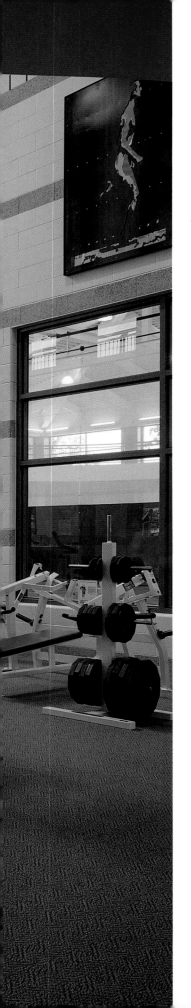

L ocated in a former cornfield in this fast-growing community just outside Columbus, the Dublin Community Recreation Center in Ohio effectively translates the latest in health club design to a suburban setting. Created by Moody/Nolan Ltd., the massive public facility offers a regional interpretation and prototype of indoor recreation as shared community activity and experience. A broad range of leisure, wellness, fitness, and sports activities accommodates patrons from preschoolers to seniors.

The architects employed shingle roofs, overhangs, wood trellises, and a palette of stone and stucco to integrate the center with its

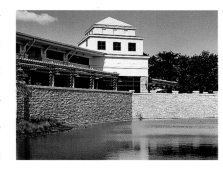

setting in a residential neighbor-hood park. A seamless transition from exterior to interior is achieved by numerous window walls, sky-lights, and glass partitions. The center is organized around a recreation lounge, flanked by the registration and control desks. Every amenity is visible from the lounge—gym, aerobics studio, track, leisure and competitive pools—to encourage their use. The mezzanine track epitomizes the interconnection of the facility, overlooking the park and all the fitness amenities in a single circuit. Vibrant yet residential purples, blues, and grays prevail, and commissioned artwork harmonizes with the architecture.

The center offers activities for all ages, and special changing rooms for families, seniors, or persons with disabilities. The building's architecture and landscaping were planned with phase two in mind: an arts center—to ensure sound minds as well as bodies.

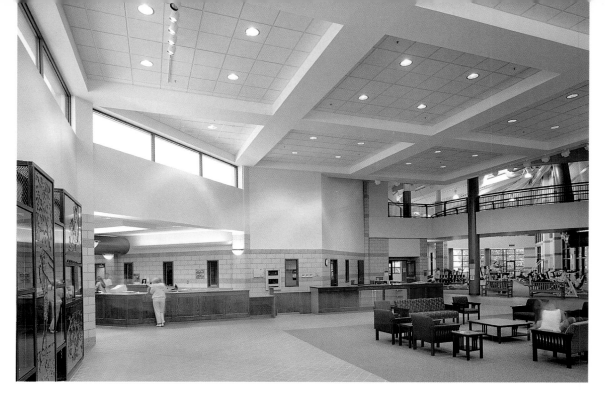

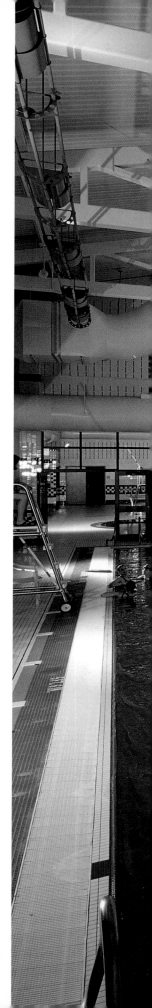

PREVIOUS SPREAD A mezzanine track provides views indoors and out. A new pond, overlooked by a sunning terrace, controls storm water and provides an alluring setting. ABOVE Every activity offered by the center is visible from the lounge to promote expanded use of the facility and encourage family use. BELOW & RIGHT The center features leisure and competitive pools, and aquatic classes for people of all ages. NEXT SPREAD Windows overlooking the basketball courts promote visual interaction.

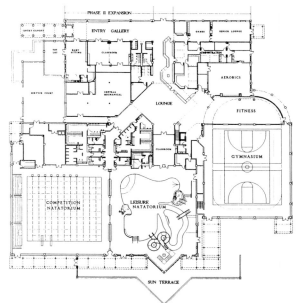

location: **Dublin, Ohio**
architect/interior designer: **Moody/Nolan Ltd., Inc.**
photographers: **© 1997 D.R. Goff;**
© Owen Smithers, LaRocco & Smithers, Inc.
square feet/meters: **90,000/8,361**
design budget: **$10 million**

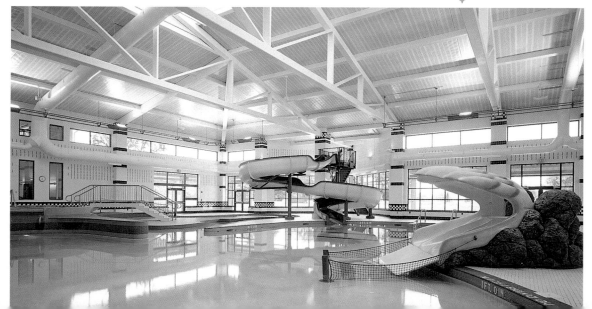

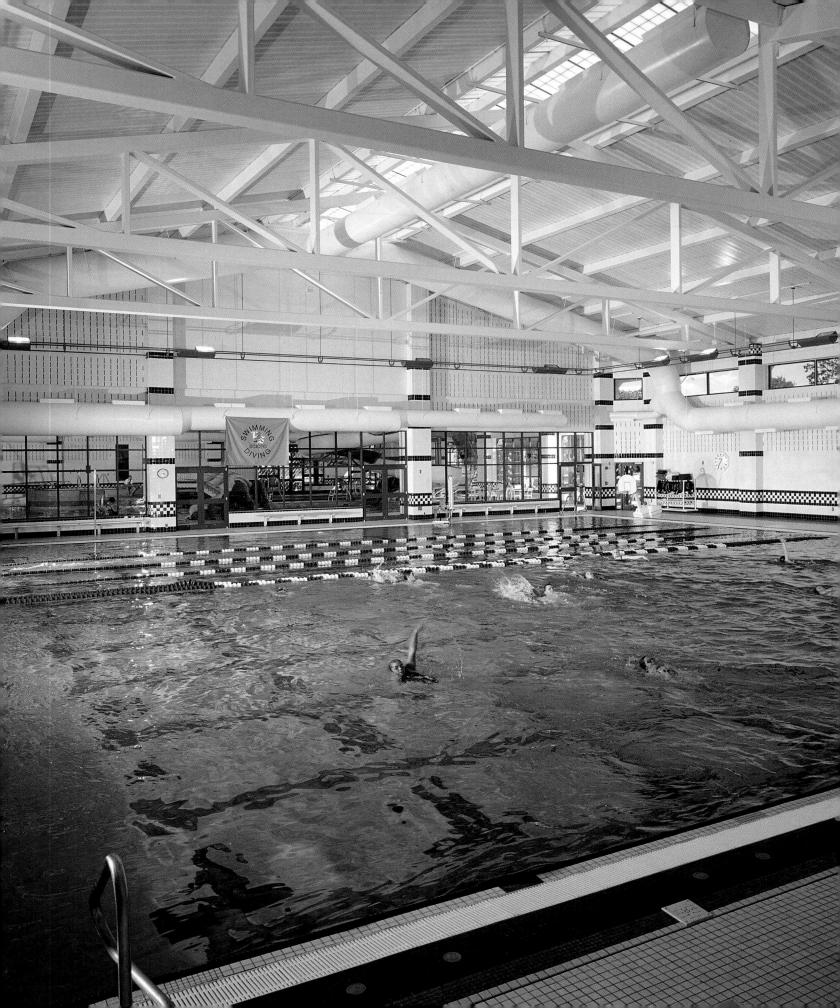

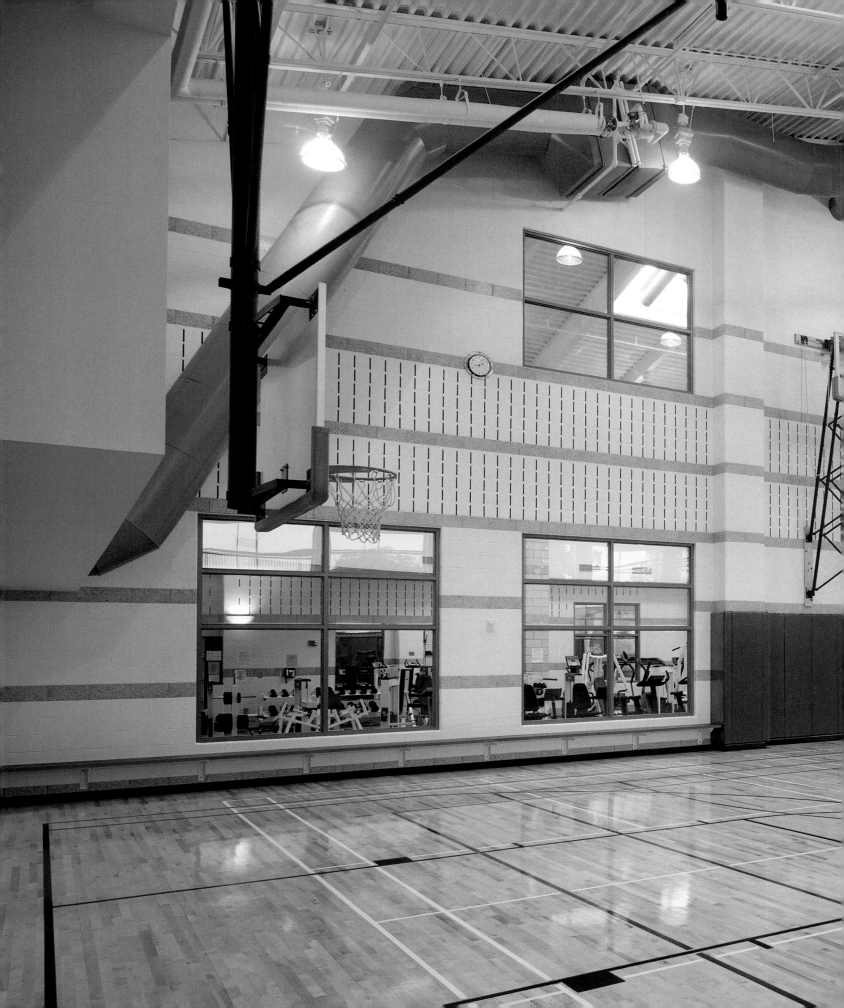

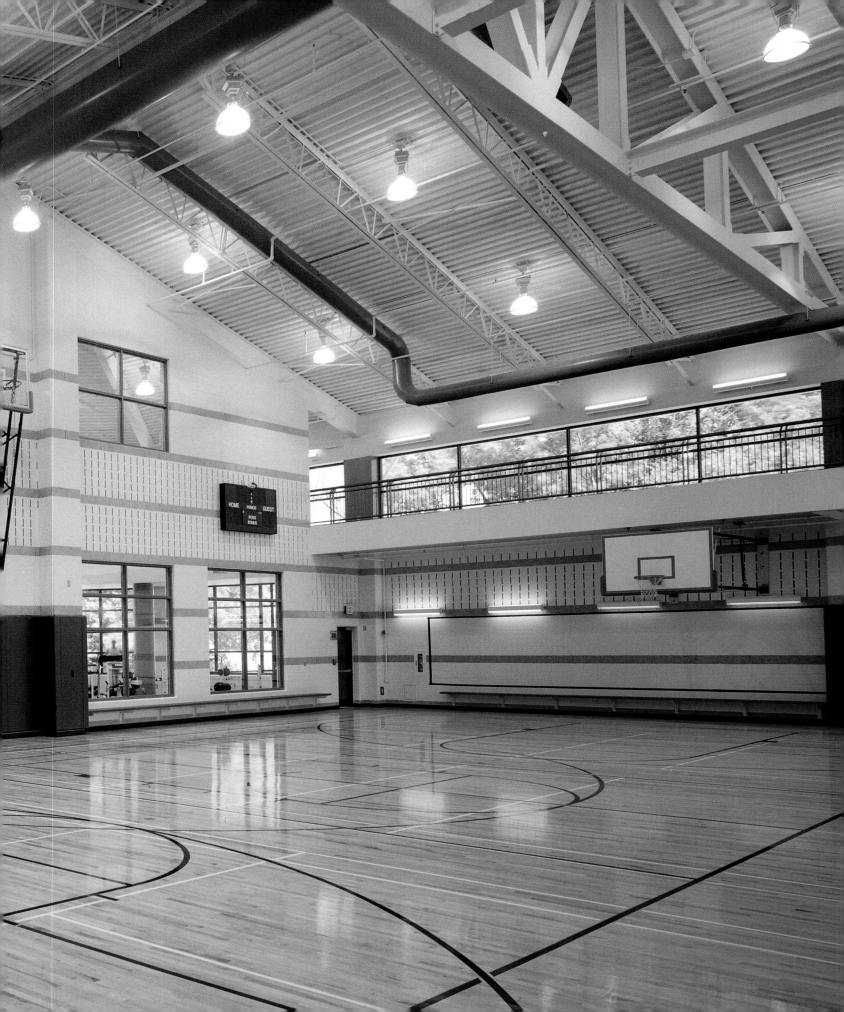

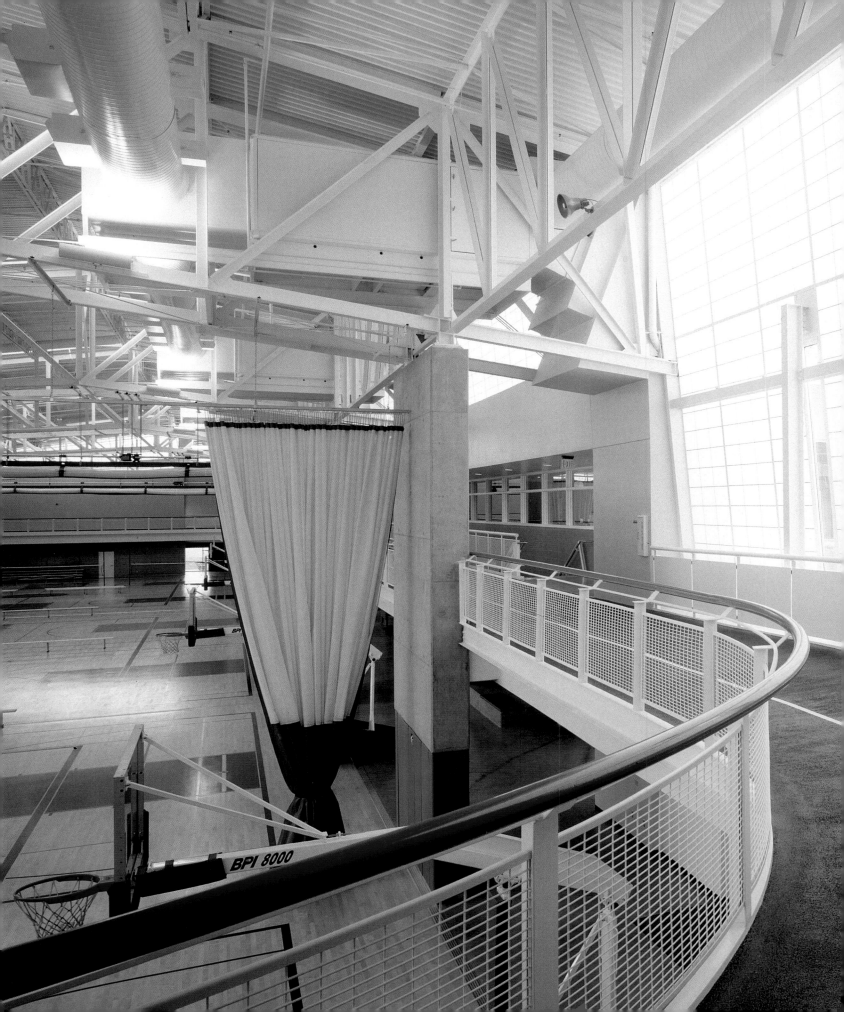

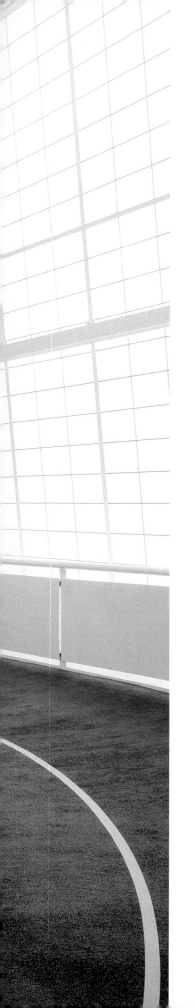

Located in the sports enthusiast city of Beaverton (home to Nike's corporate headquarters), the 66-acre Tualatin Hills Parks and Recreation District campus in Oregon is one of the Northwest's largest. Comprised of playing fields, aquatics, and tennis facilities, its success has led to the addition of an athletic center, created by BOORA Architects, Inc.

Set on former farmland, the building was conceived as an earthwork in an effort to connect to the region's agrarian roots. The perimeter berms on three sides of the Great Hall gracefully reduce the scale of the structure and blend it into the slope of the land. The upper level lobby, check-in desk, and offices overlook both interior and exterior courts to aid supervision. The interior houses

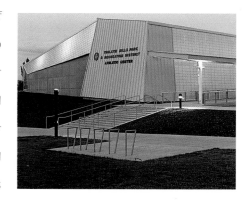

basketball, volleyball, and badminton courts, track, concessions, and a daycare/seminar room. Outside are lighted basketball courts, a soccer control shelter, and bleacher seating for 500.

The architects strove to energize the field house by emphasizing daylight, exposed construction, and architecture inspired by physical strength. The standing-seam metal walls and roof are shaped and detailed to be an extension of the land and to recall the farm buildings of the past. The white-dominated interior is accented by primary colors; indirect lighting minimizes glare. Natural light streams in through clerestory and north-facing windows that allow panoramic views from the elevated track to the fields and foothills beyond.

TUALATIN HILLS ATHLETIC CENTER

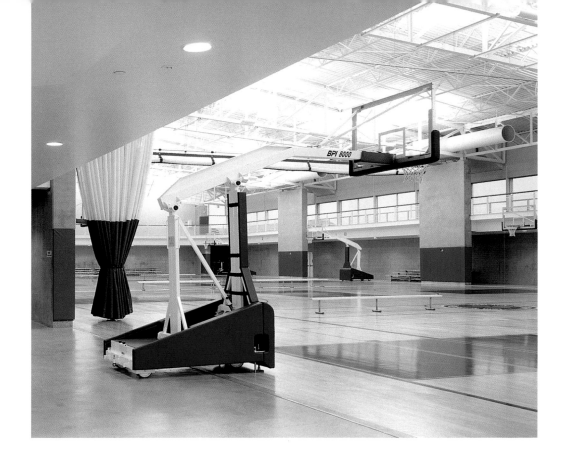

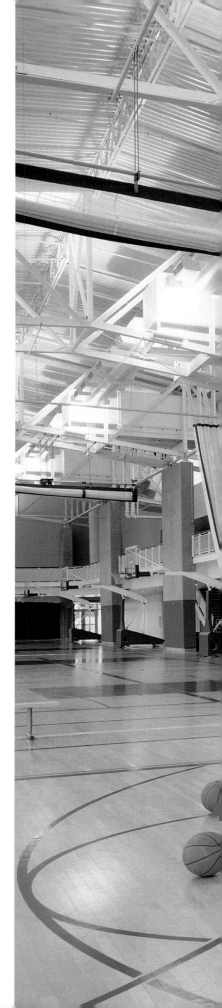

PREVIOUS SPREAD & ABOVE The forms, industrial materials, and clarity of structural expression combine the vernacular of prefabricated farm buildings with the framework of the field house. RIGHT In the Great Hall, concrete piers aligned with paired trusses establish the structural bays and zones for skylights and mechanical units, and reinforce the boundaries of each court. An elevated track overlooks the basketball courts.

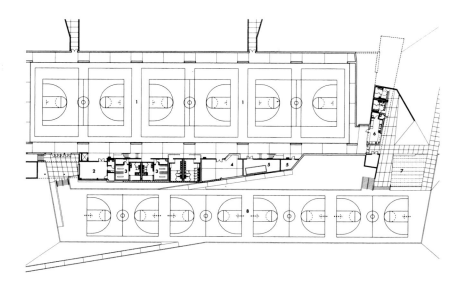

location: Beaverton, Oregon
architect/interior designer: BOORA Architects, Inc.
photographer: John Hughel, Portland, Oregon
square feet/meters: 60,027/5,577
design budget: $6 million

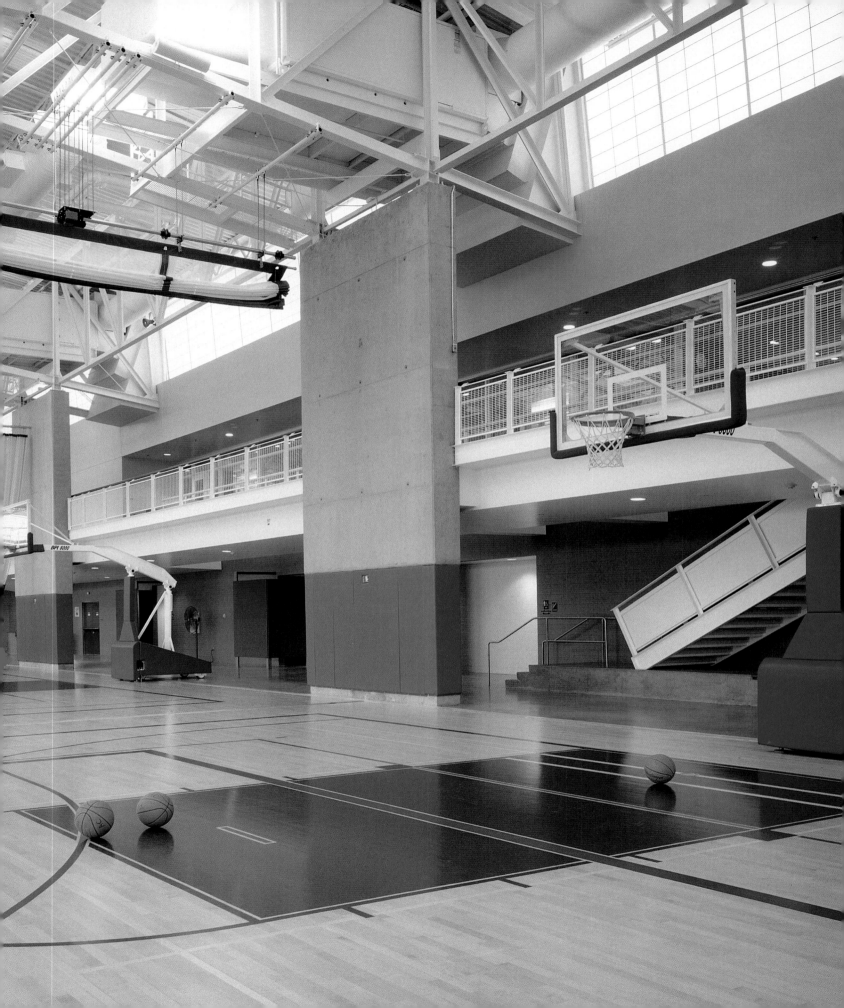

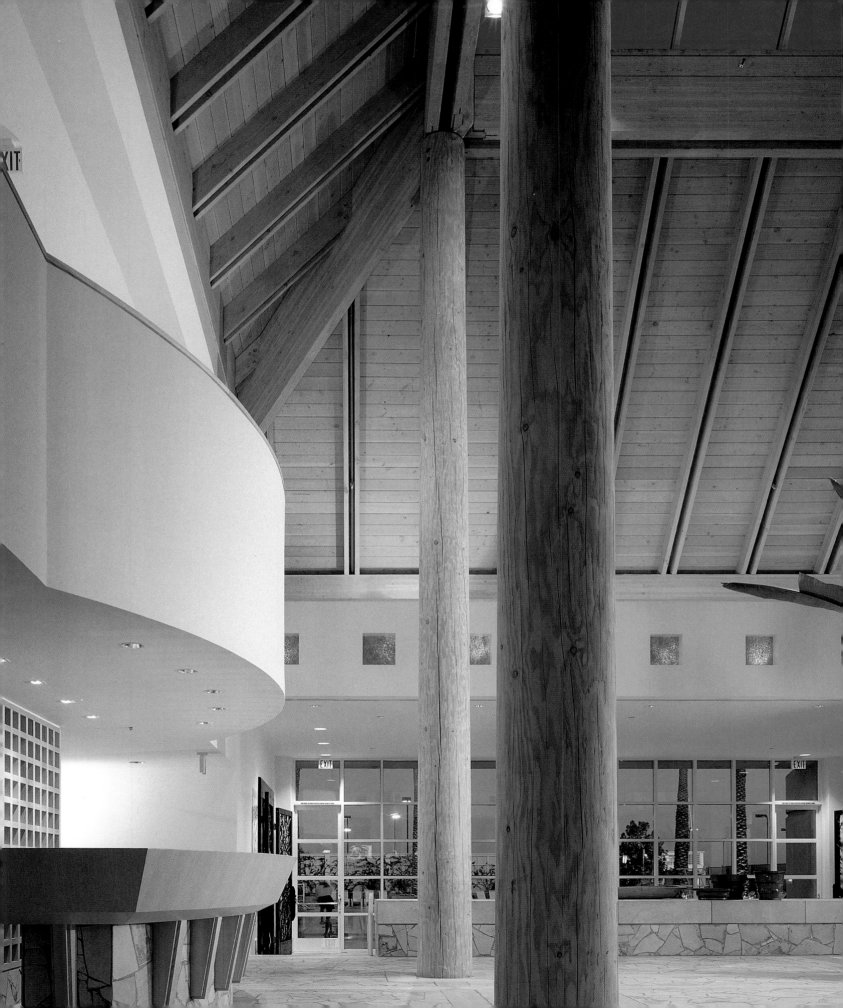

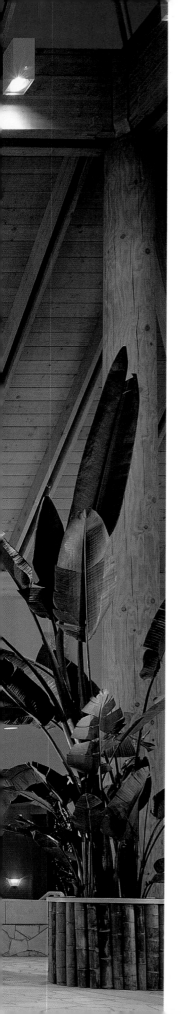

The sixth location operated by Western Athletic Clubs, the Pacific Athletic Club opened in 1992 with a fully subscribed membership and a waiting list. Situated on almost ten acres in suburban Redwood City, California, the sprawling facility lives up to the promise of a sports "resort." A wealth of offerings includes a basketball gym, indoor and outdoor tennis courts, a lap pool, recreational pool and outdoor spa, children's wading pool, squash courts, and an 8,500-square-foot, fully loaded fitness center.

Since the owners believe that each of their clubs should cater to the community it serves, the interiors by Orlando Diaz-Azcuy Designs support the upscale yet relaxed and family-friendly needs of its members. Specialized facilities meet the club's goal to be everything to everyone with family programming which includes a child-care center and enclosed playground. Dining and socializing are enjoyed in a 175-seat dining 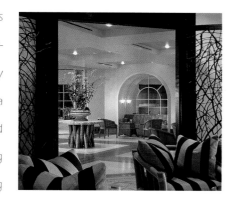 room, cafe, private meeting rooms, and an outdoor dining courtyard. Other amenities include a women's workout area, executive locker rooms, and the Sanctuary—a massage and beauty spa. Materials are sampled from the California landscape; wood is used in abundance, often untreated, for soaring ceilings and columns, custom furniture, and decorative accents. Light streams through skylights and windows. Social spaces achieve the ambiance of a four-star resort, with residential-style furniture of high-end materials and fabrics. Workout spaces are finished in natural colors, with vistas of the outdoor facilities and famous redwood trees.

PACIFIC ATHLETIC CLUB

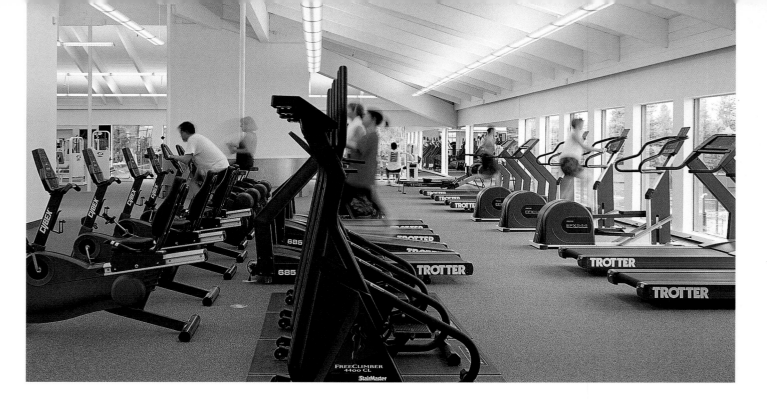

PREVIOUS SPREAD Tree trunk columns in the skylit atrium support a pitched roof of wood beams and slats. Pacific Athletic Club offers a variety of spaces for socializing; upholstered chairs and coffee tables encourage lingering. ABOVE Members using cardiovascular equipment can choose to watch a number of televisions or face the views outdoors. RIGHT The fitness center contains a complex Cybex weight training circuit and extensive cardiovascular equipment. BELOW The 175-seat dining room features double-height ceilings, comfortable furniture, and decorative murals for a clubhouse atmosphere. In its quest to branch out to the community, the club opens its dining and spa facilities to nonmembers. OPPOSITE The circuit training area is oriented toward the outdoor tennis courts through floor-to-ceiling windows which add visual variety.

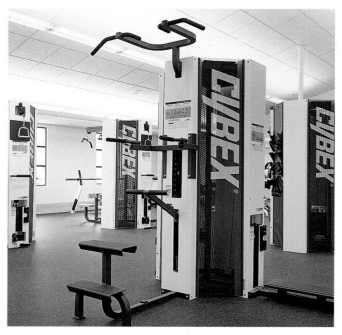

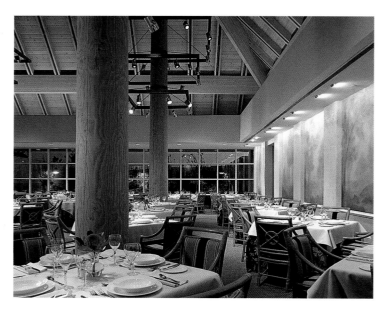

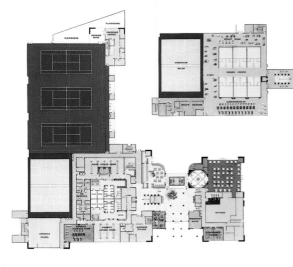

location: Redwood City, California
architect: DES Architects + Engineers
interior designer: Orlando Diaz-Azcuy Designs, Inc.
photographers: Nick Merrick/Hedrich Blessing; © John Sutton 1998
square feet/meters: 86,000/7,989
design budget: not disclosed

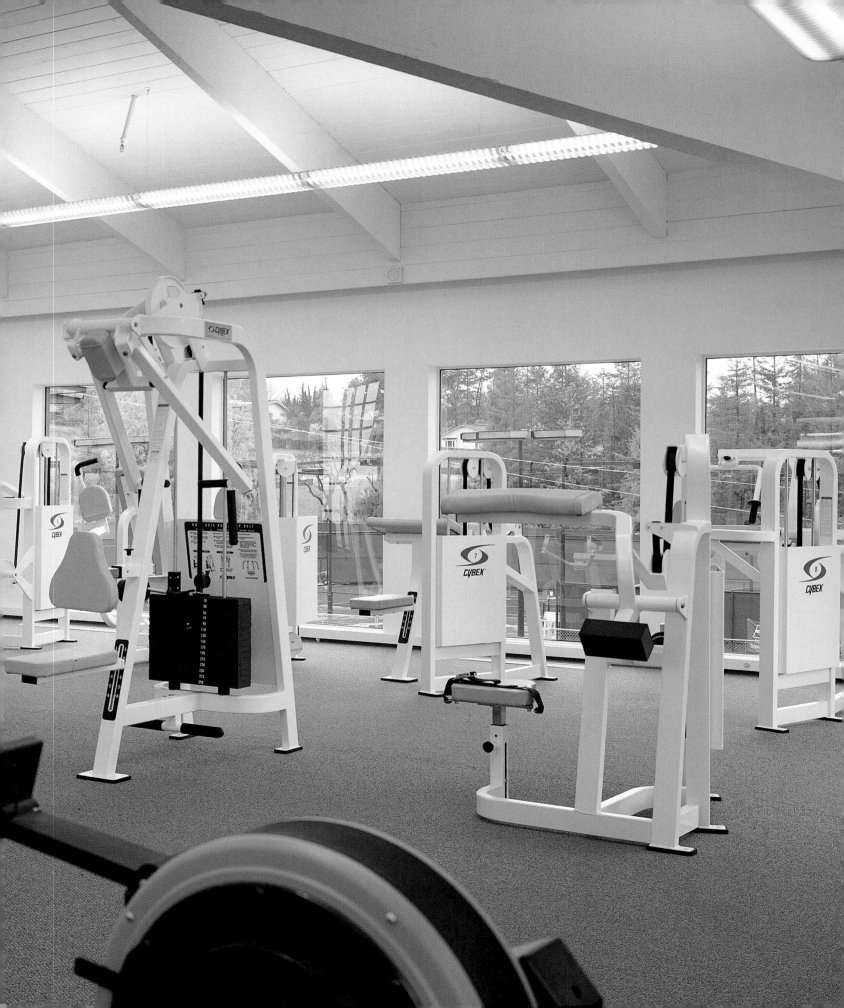

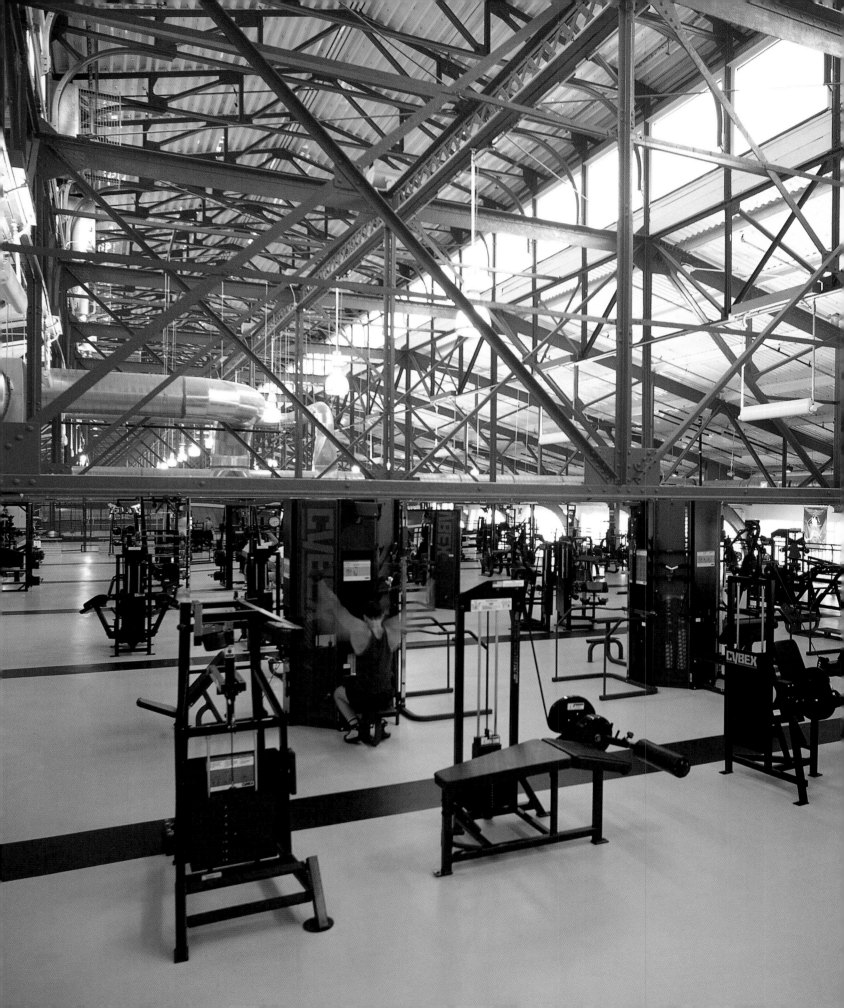

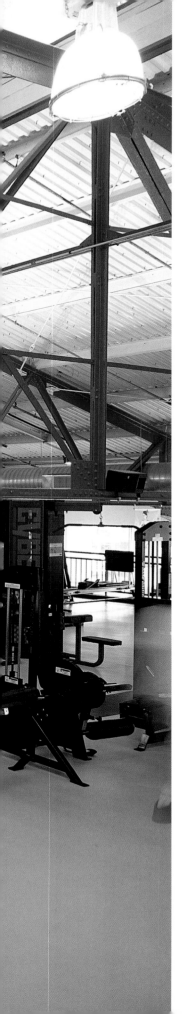

When plans were announced to create a sports center on four neglected piers on the Hudson River, many Manhattanites were skeptical. Both the investors and Butler Rogers Baskett Architects knew that Chelsea Piers, not easily accessible to most New Yorkers, would have to be well worth the trip. Market research of the area's current offerings determined the program: indoor and outdoor hockey, gymnastics, skateboarding, rollerskating, and basketball facilities (among others) were added to a golf driving range and health club. Constructed in 1910 as passenger terminals for the luxury liners of that era, today Chelsea Piers is a bustling complex, offering summer camps, sports leagues, television and movie production, and special events.

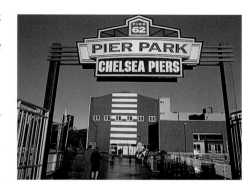

The massive Sports Center on Pier 60 is a light-filled, amenity-packed extravaganza. "We wanted it to be open, with great views," says project manager Laurence Marner. The architects installed windows and skylights, and exploited the lofty ceilings and 650-foot-long space. More than 20,000 square feet of cardiovascular and strength training equipment, and aerobics studios is just the beginning: the center offers the world's longest indoor running track and the largest rock climbing wall in the Northeast. The 18,000-square-foot flexible infield embodies a 2,000-seat arena which houses track-and-field events, indoor sand volleyball and touch football, basketball courts, and a boxing ring. The riverfront pool sports a stunning 6,000-square-foot outdoor sundeck. Other perks include saunas, steam rooms, a sports medicine and performance center, food court, and beauty spa.

THE SPORTS CENTER AT CHELSEA PIERS

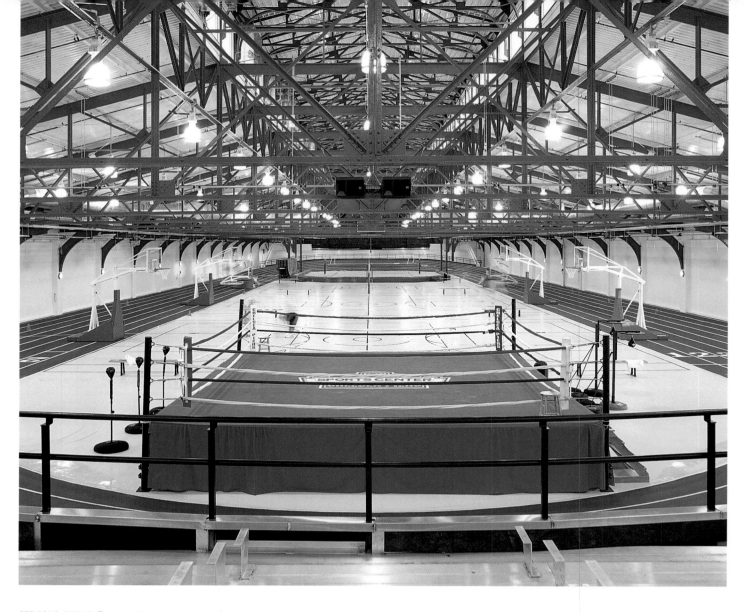

PREVIOUS SPREAD Twenty-thousand square feet of cardiovascular, circuit, and strength training equipment are housed mainly on the Sports Center's second floor, under the original trusses and lofty ceilings of the former passenger terminal. ABOVE The 18,000-square-foot flexible infield houses basketball courts, a boxing ring, and the world's longest indoor running track. BELOW LEFT & RIGHT The six-lane, banked rubber track is used for both recreation and competition. OPPOSITE The 45-foot-high climbing wall is the largest in the Northeast; climbing equipment is available for sale or rent at an adjacent store.

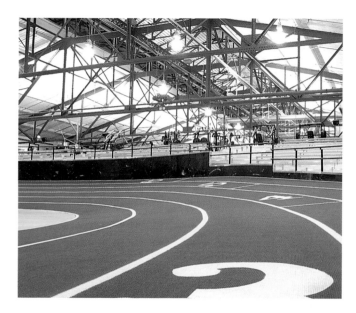

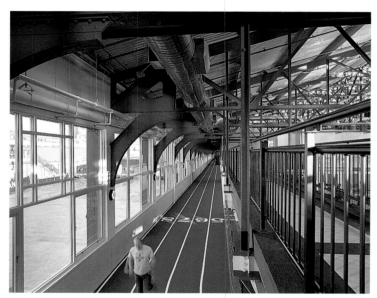

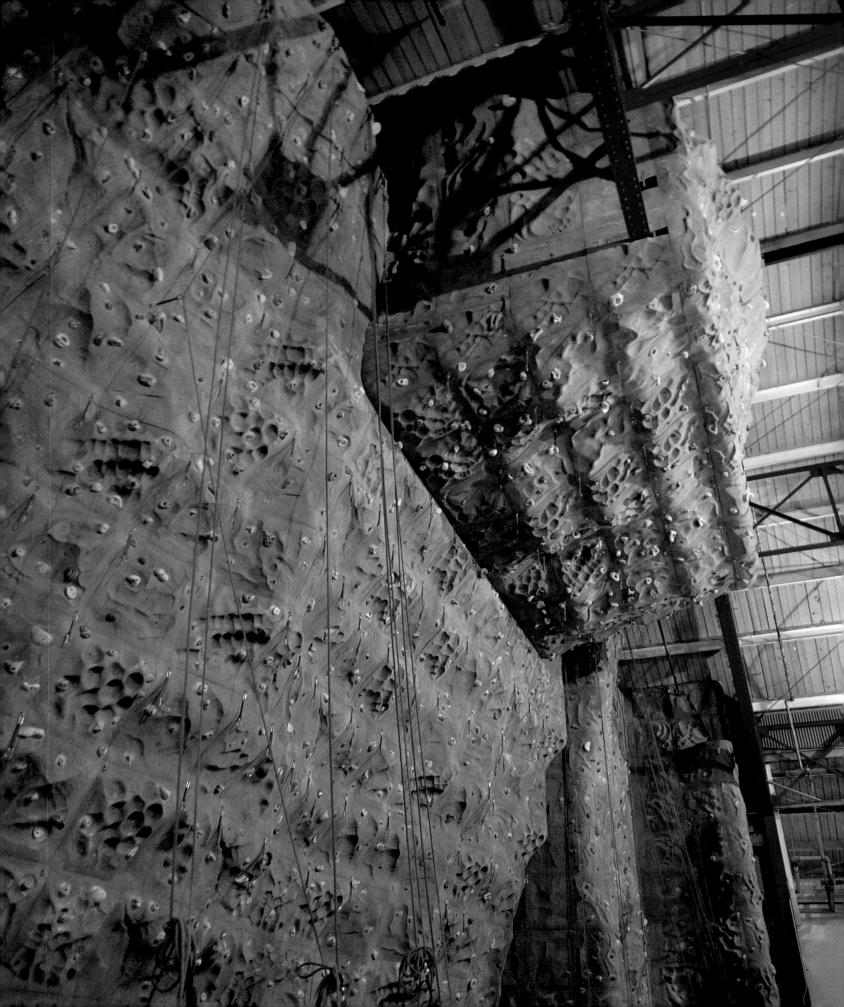

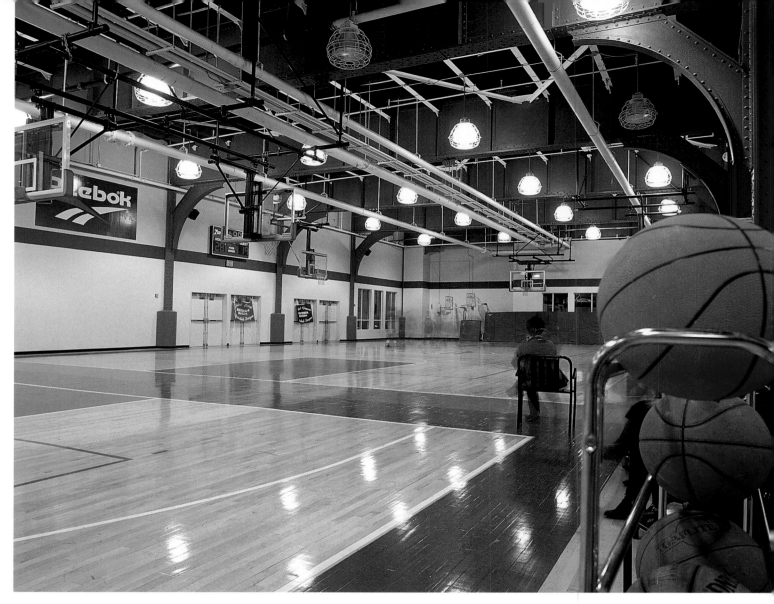

location: New York, New York
architect/interior designer: Butler Rogers Baskett Architects
photographer: Fred George Photography
square feet/meters: 119,000/11,055
design budget: $12.5 million
club membership: 3,500

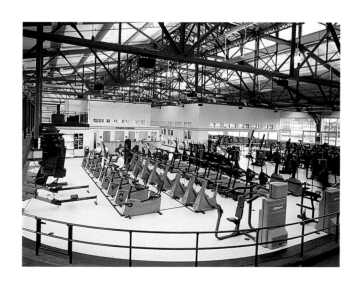

61

60

59

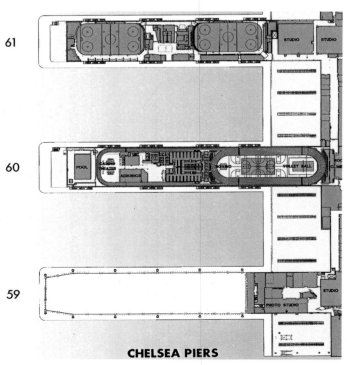

CHELSEA PIERS

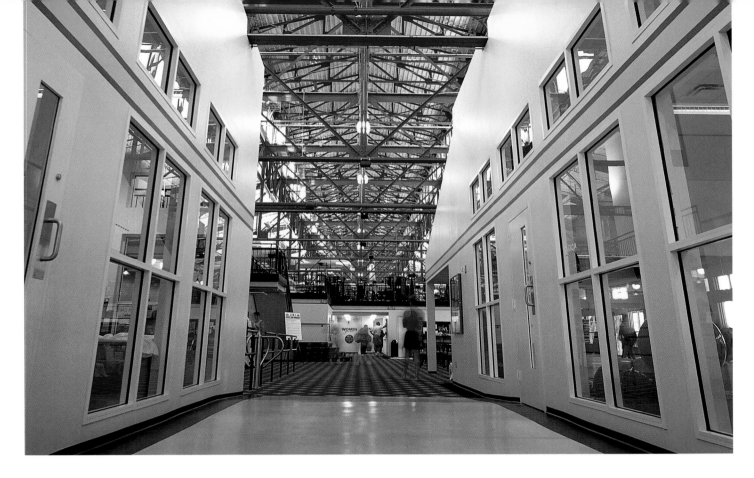

OPPOSITE ABOVE The dimensions of Chelsea Piers provided an ideal setting for basketball courts. Lighting is suspended from the immense ceiling height. OPPOSITE BELOW Cardiovascular equipment is sited on the first floor, adjacent to the aerobics studios. ABOVE Two windowed studios totaling 4,000 square feet are dedicated to aerobics. BELOW The 25-yard indoor pool and whirlpool overlook the 6,000-square-foot sundeck on the Hudson River—complete with outdoor shower.

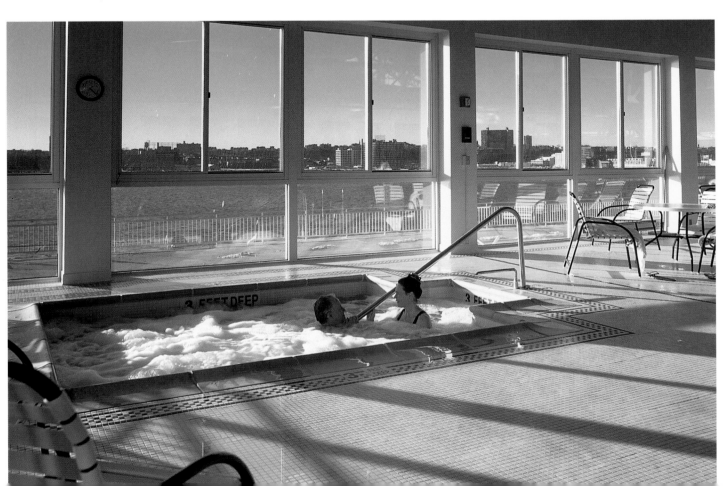

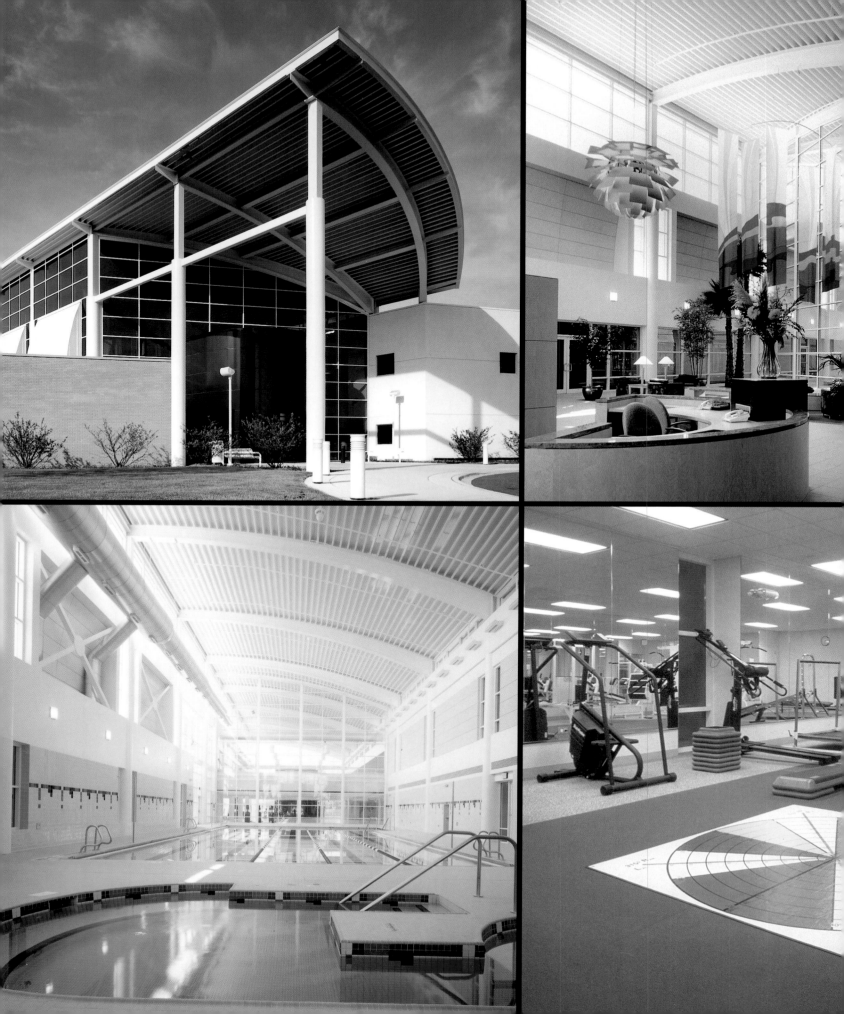

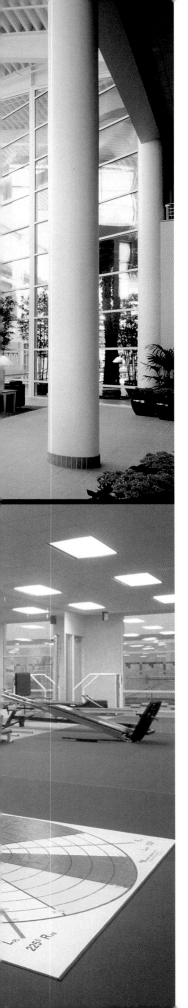

The Northwest Community Hospital Wellness Center provides a balance of fitness and medical programs focused not only on healing but on prevention and education. To create an atmosphere of vigor and health, OWP&P Architects juxtaposed the orthogonal form of the International Style against the organic shapes of nature. The design revolves around a three-story glass spine which runs the length of the building and admits natural light while interconnecting the main spaces.

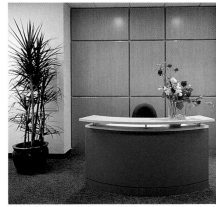

The center is divided into fitness, clinical outpatient, and community service components. On the first floor are the physical medicine and rehabilitation clinic, control desk, locker rooms, lap pool, equipment floor, aerobics studio, and running track; community services are on the second floor. To provide motivation to those entering the facility, all activities within are visible from the spacious double-height lobby (which is oversized to accommodate users in wheelchairs). The five banner colors in the entranceway correlate to the departments and establish pathways in the matching carpeting and reception stations of colored stained wood. Since the hospital required a building that could be expanded in the future, the architects chose flexible materials, such as a steel frame with a composite metal deck, glass, and light construction partitions. Sessions held with neighbors to listen to concerns they had regarding the building program and its impact on the neighborhood, helps to account for the center's resounding success.

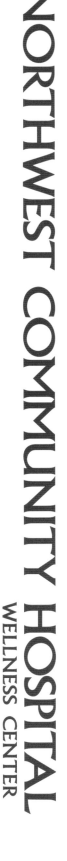

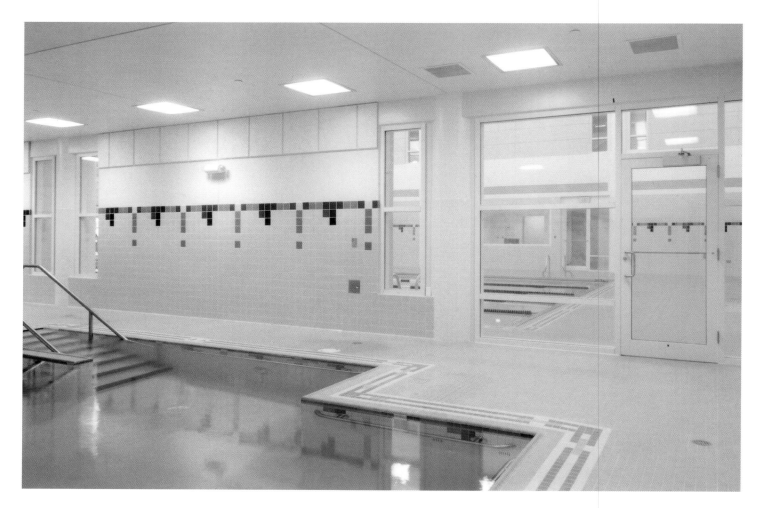

PREVIOUS SPREAD The lobby creates an open feeling and allows patients in wheelchairs or on crutches to maneuver easily. The bold colors in the exercise areas are borrowed from the entranceway banners and continue throughout the center. Glass, masonry and painted metal tie the building into the context of the hospital campus. ABOVE Interconnecting spaces such as those in the pool area provide motivation through the visibility of other users exercising. RIGHT The second floor, accessible from the lobby staircase, is devoted to community activities, such as health education classes and meetings. OPPOSITE ABOVE Bold, soaring architecture promotes a feeling of spaciousness, health, and brightness. OPPOSITE BELOW Spacious locker rooms accommodate both member and patient users.

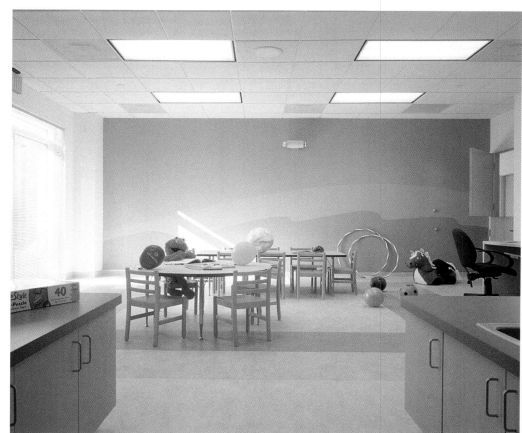

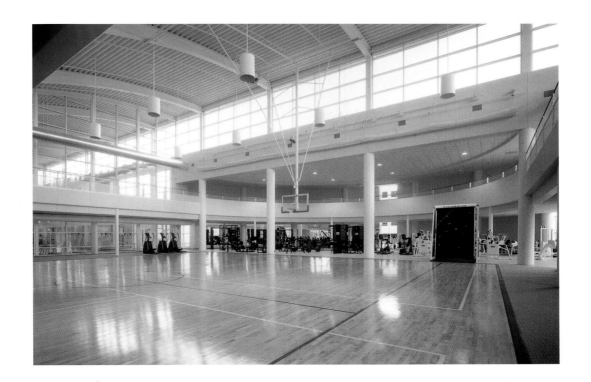

location: **Arlington Heights, Illinois**
architect/interior designer: **OWP&P Architects, Inc.**
photographer: **Paul Schlismann Photography**
square feet/meters: **85,000/7,897**
design budget: **$13 million**
club membership: **3,200**

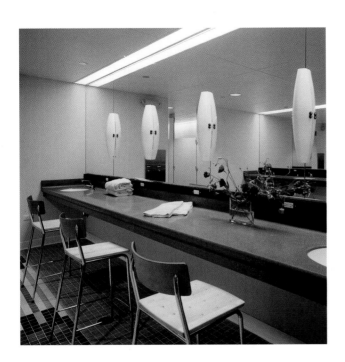

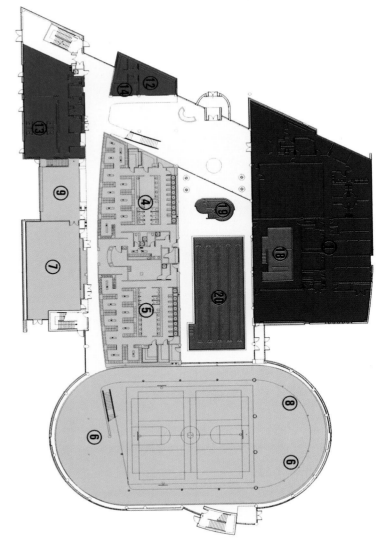

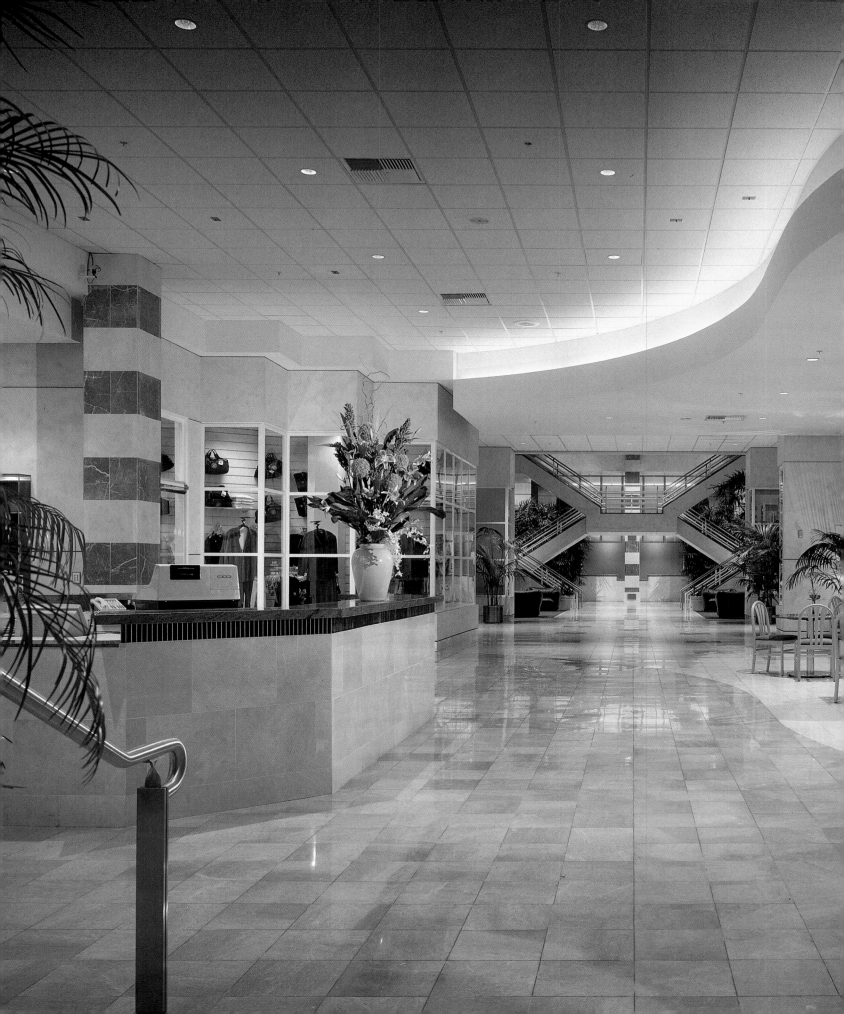

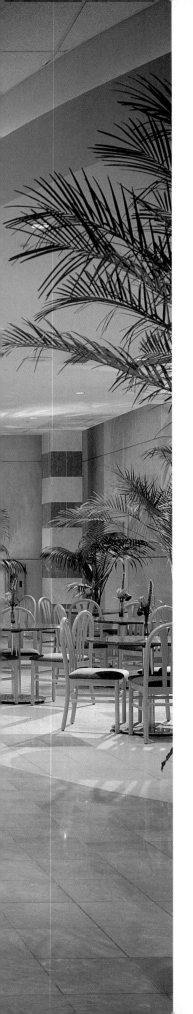

The Sports Club Company creates urban country clubs—sprawling spaces with unlimited amenities and resort-like interiors. Hair and body salons, restaurants, and cafés are sited alongside the abundant sports facilities, allowing a member to "escape for an hour or the whole day," says Kent Walker, interior designer. The California locations include the Sports Club/LA which had been destroyed in an earthquake; and the Sports Club/Irvine. Most recently, Reebok Sports Club/NY was installed in Manhattan, a joint venture with Reebok.

Each club builds on the successes of previous clubs, and reflects new trends and its location. The first two are pure southern California: sunlight, indoor-outdoor spaces, and tropical colors and materials. The Irvine 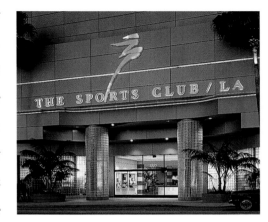 club has a soaring atrium, while the Los Angeles club has valet parking and a cruise ship-scale marble concourse. Both feature grand staircases from which to see and be seen. When the designs for the New York club were thought too "West Coast," the designer introduced a subtle, urban edge. Whereas the first gyms employ pale wood, skin-flattering tans and pinks, a palette of darker tones such as charcoal gray and silver was created for New York, using a transitional gray-purple.

Certain programming concepts are observed: the dining areas flow into the main circulation space, creating a sense of conviviality.

THE SPORTS CLUBS

Cardiovascular equipment is located near the atrium and basketball courts. Flexibility is key—since new activities and equipment proliferate, the use of space is constantly reevaluated. Materials convey casual elegance, with a simple yet high-end palette that can withstand the traffic of over a thousand members a day. Maintenance is of prime importance, as Walker explains, "The materials are the background; the members are the focus."

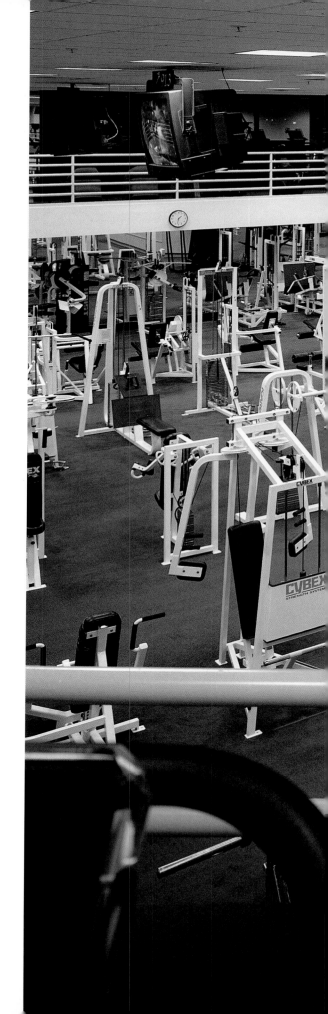

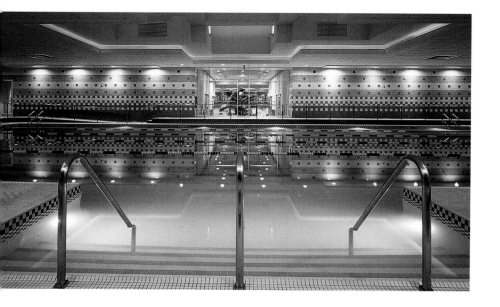

The Sports Club/LA

PREVIOUS SPREAD Retail and café spaces in the Los Angeles club's grand concourse are part of the cruise ship-inspired program, and are sited to attract members on their way to work out. The entrance glows with neon detailing and backlit glass block walls. **ABOVE** The pool is finished in signature West Coast detailing: pastels and bright colors (flattering to skin tones), with a view to palm trees on the level below. **RIGHT** A mezzanine level of cardiovascular equipment offers visual variety through large televisions and a view to the strength training area below.

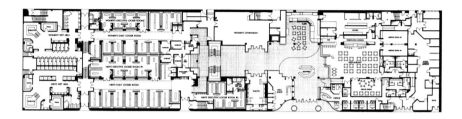

location: **Los Angeles, California**
architect: **Langdon Wilson Architecture Planning**
interior designer: **J. Kent Walker Design**
photographer: **Milroy & McAleer Photography**
square feet/meters: **100,000/9,290**
design budget: **not disclosed**
club membership: **10,000**

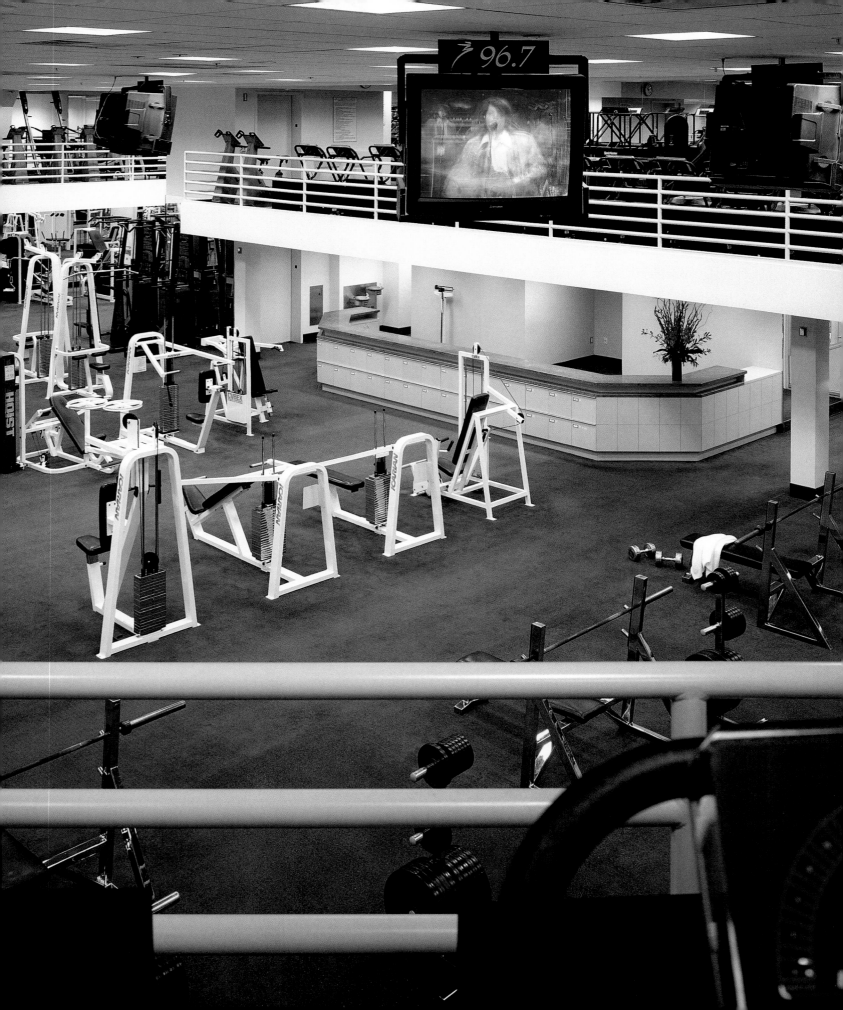

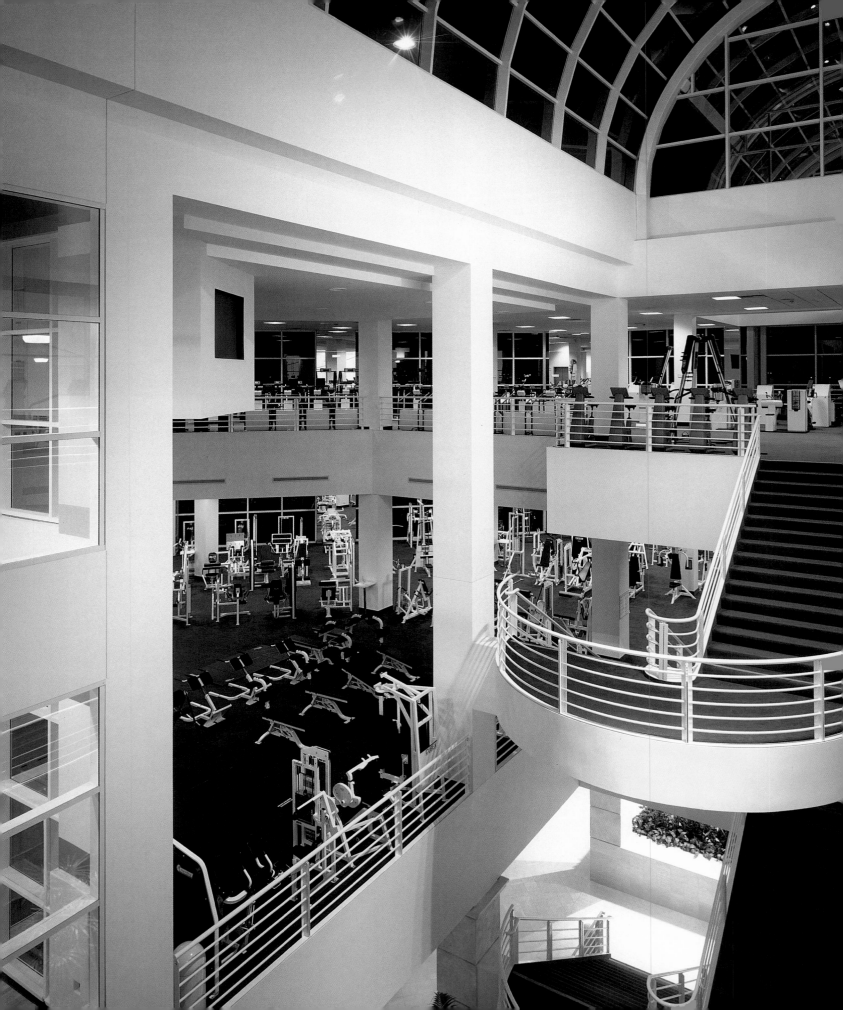

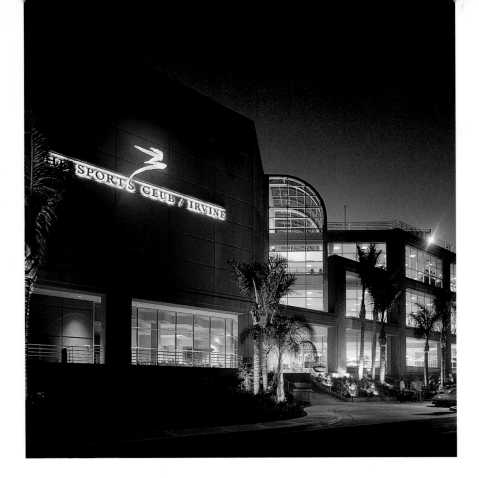

The Sports Club/Irvine

OPPOSITE The grand staircase is common to all the Sports Clubs' gyms, creating a social center and visual invitation to the club's numerous offerings. **LEFT** The exterior of the Irvine club is inviting, featuring resort-inspired steps and landscaping and floor-to-ceiling glass panels and atrium. **BELOW LEFT** In the basketball courts, decoration is kept to a minimum, with subtle pastel striping, and glass windows for interested passersby.

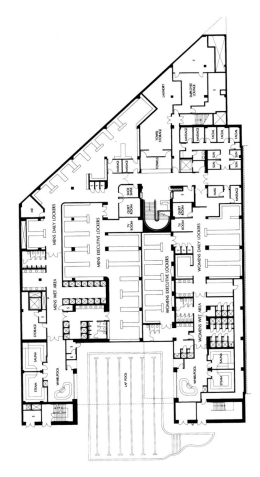

location: **Irvine, California**
architect: **Langdon Wilson Architecture Planning**
interior designer: **J. Kent Walker Design**
photographer: **Milroy & McAleer Photography**
square feet/meters: **130,000/12,077**
design budget: **not disclosed**
club membership: **10,000**

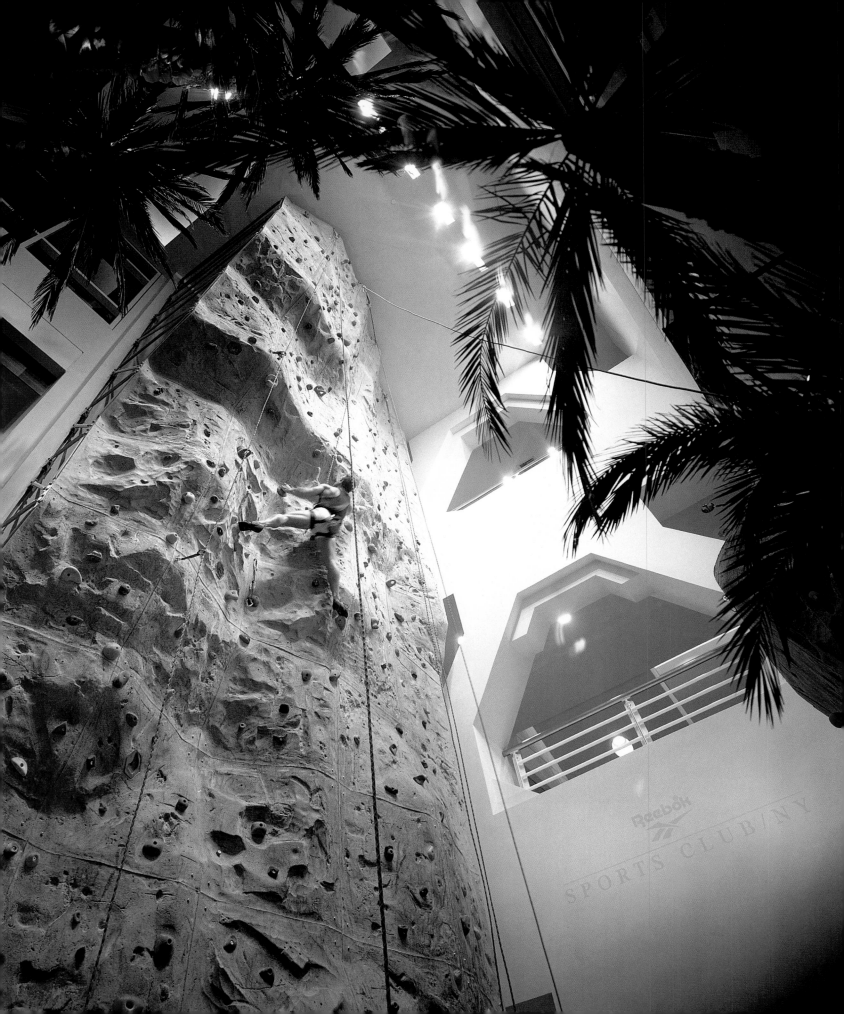

Reebok Sports Club/NY

OPPOSITE A dramatic climbing wall rises three stories, serving as both a diversion for club members and an attraction for visitors. BELOW The lobby of the New York club has the aura of a fine hotel, with comfortable reception and dining areas, featuring patterned rugs, wood paneling, and paintings. RIGHT The signature atrium overlooks the cardiovascular area; palm trees are reminiscent of the California clubs. The dark blue carpet is in contrast to the pastels of the West coast palette. BELOW RIGHT The pool area is characterized by natural light and views; colorful tiles add warmth. BOTTOM The palette of the New York club replaces the sunny California colors with cool tones of silvery gray, plum, and apricot.

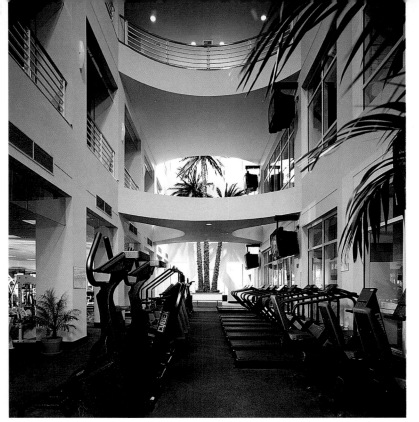

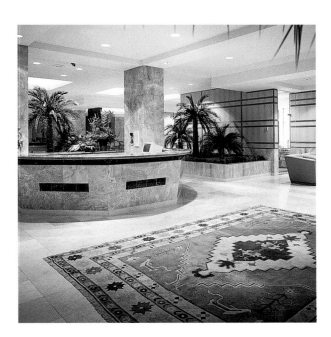

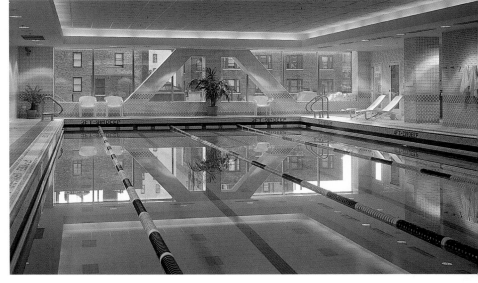

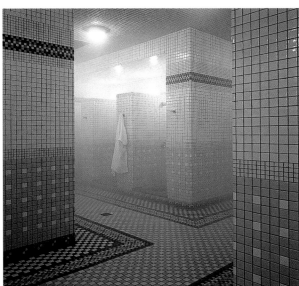

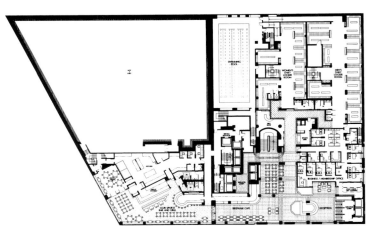

location: **New York, New York**
architect: **Langdon Wilson Architecture Planning**
interior designer: **J. Kent Walker Design**
photographer: **Milroy & McAleer Photography**
square feet/meters: **140,000/13,006**
design budget: **not disclosed**
club membership: **10,000**

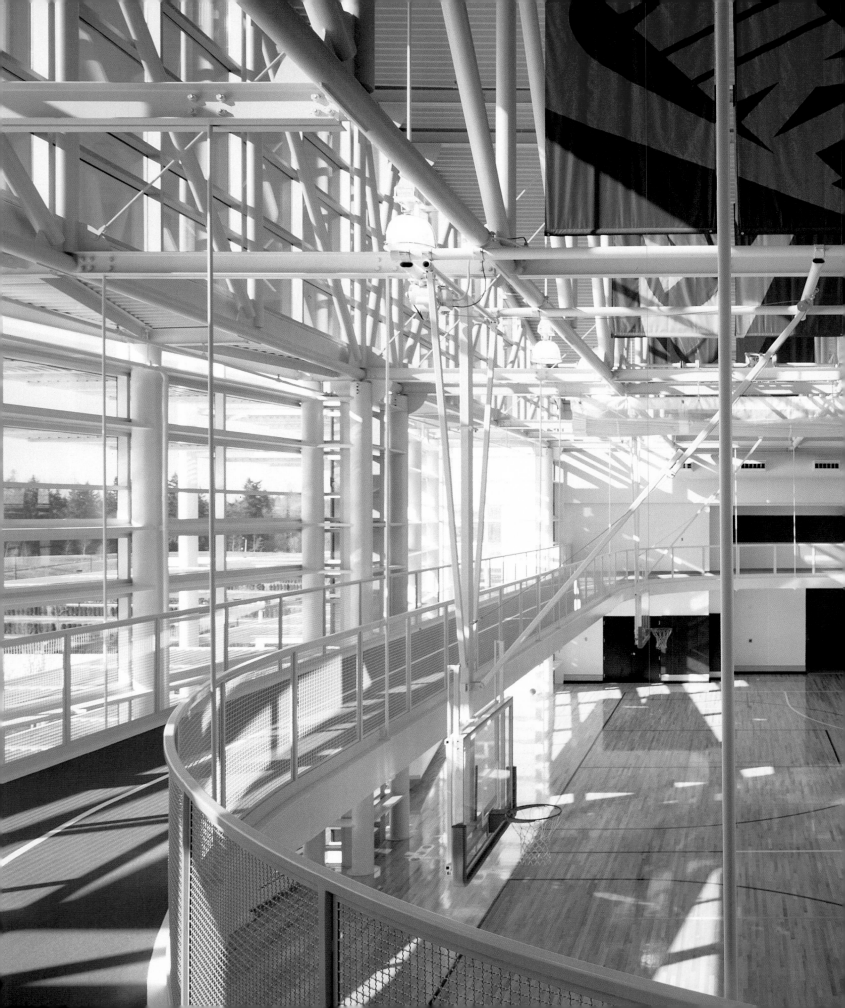

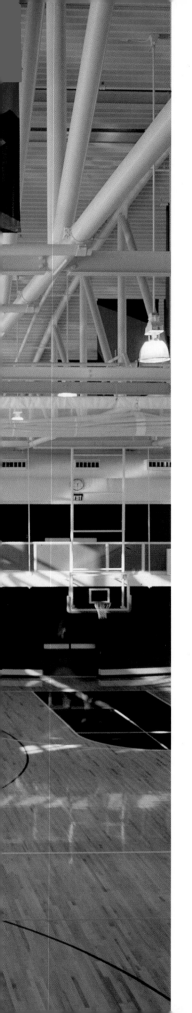

Situated on the 74-acre wooded Nike corporate campus, the Bo Jackson Sports & Fitness Center was designed as a corporate training and product testing center for use by employees and athletes involved in footwear and apparel development. The priorities of Nike and TVA Architects centered on creating an environment informed by high standards in athleticism. In this state-of-the-art facility, world-class athletes could maximize personal goals. Used by visiting National Basketball Association (NBA) teams, the center was also intended to serve as the living room or social hub of the campus.

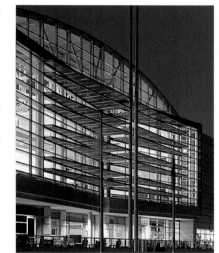

The architects employed natural light in the three-story structure as the main architectural and thematic element, to recall sandlot athletics and quintessential pick-up games in the park. The skin on the north and south elevations of the upper two stories is glass, with light diffused on the south through a series of screened fins on the exterior. The gym's north side faces offices in the adjacent building, where product designers can glance out their window to see their work in action. The ground floor houses the building entry, locker rooms, child care, and fitness institute, where users can monitor everything from body fat to blood pressure. After workouts, people gather on level two which also houses the corporate lounge, aerobic rooms, and weight rooms. Level three contains the gym, racquetball and squash courts, and running track.

BO JACKSON SPORTS & FITNESS CENTER

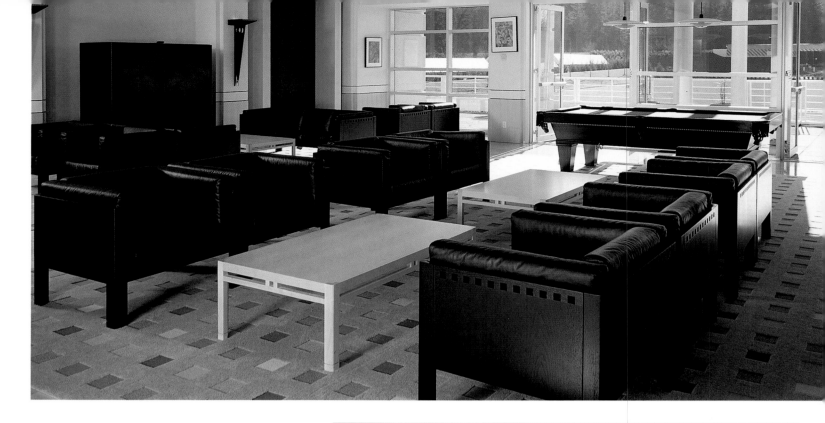

PREVIOUS SPREAD The indoor running track encircles the gym. The south face of the building is glass, with sunlight diffused through a series of screened metal fins. ABOVE One of the goals of the center was to create a social hub for Nike employees; living room-style spaces encourage informal gathering. RIGHT Black-and-white photography depicts the center's namesake. OPPOSITE ABOVE LEFT Simple yet high-end locker rooms employ elements such as wood, glass, and metal mesh. OPPOSITE ABOVE RIGHT Outdoor tennis courts are one of various amenities, providing visual stimulation to product designers walking through the campus. OPPOSITE BELOW The gym is contained within a "glass room," visually connecting it to the fields and woods beyond. NEXT SPREAD Custom light fixtures recall Olympic torches.

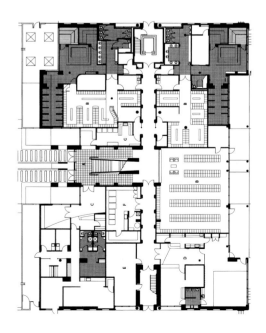

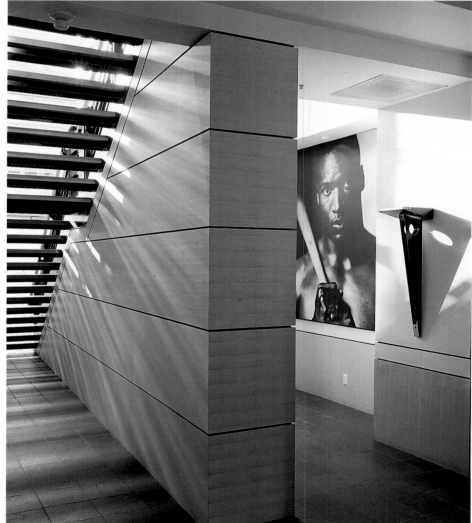

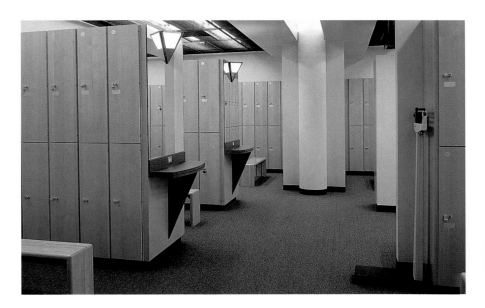

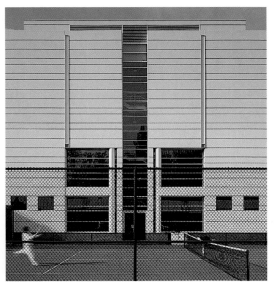

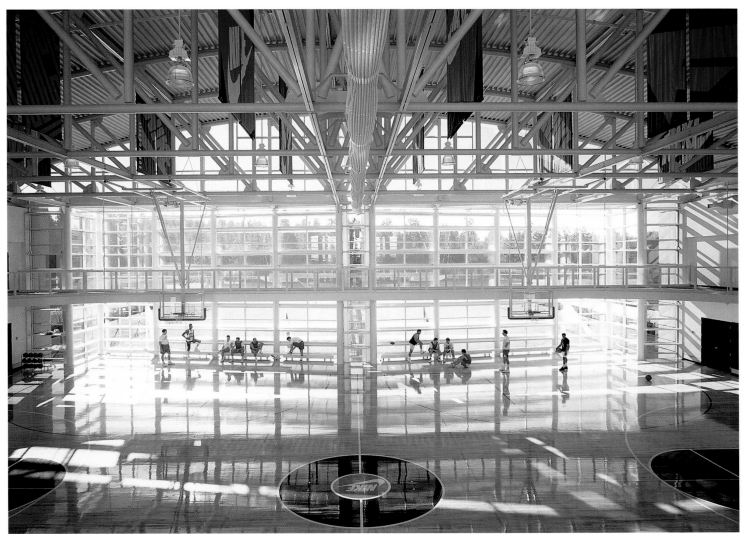

location: **Beaverton, Oregon**
architect/interior designer: **TVA Architects**
photographers: © **Richard Barnes; Strode Photographic LLC**
square feet/meters: **60,000/5,574**
design budget: **$7 million**
club membership: **1,200**

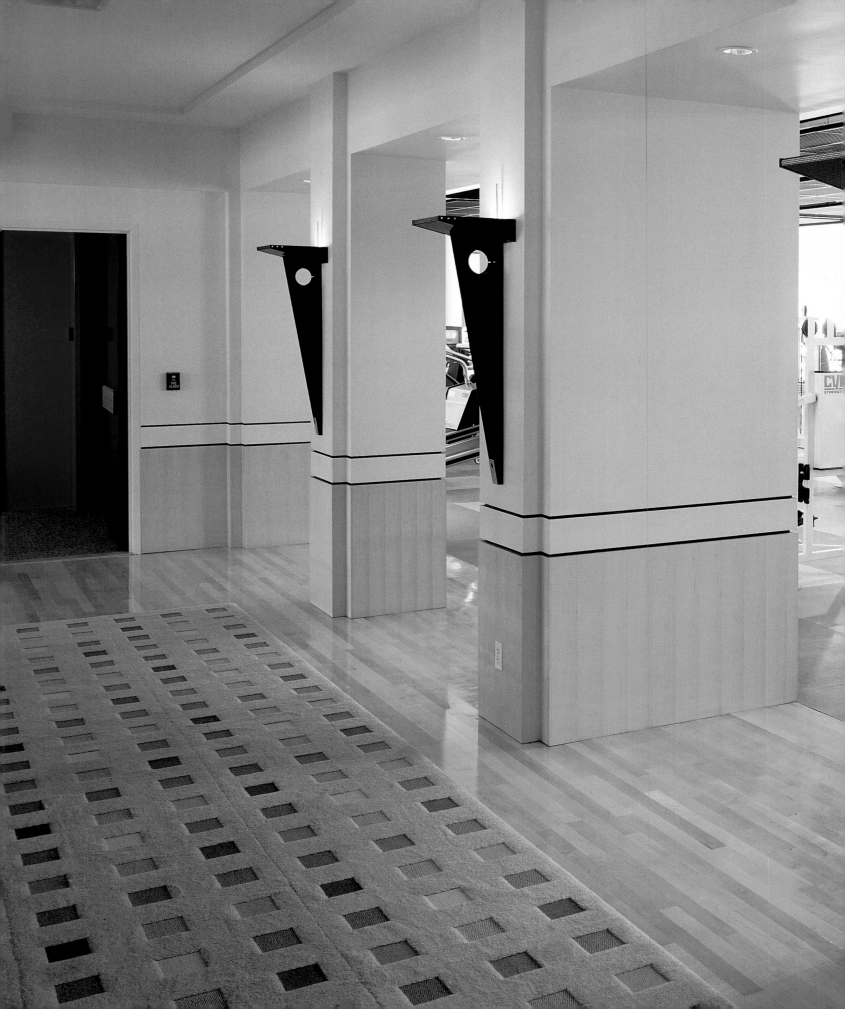

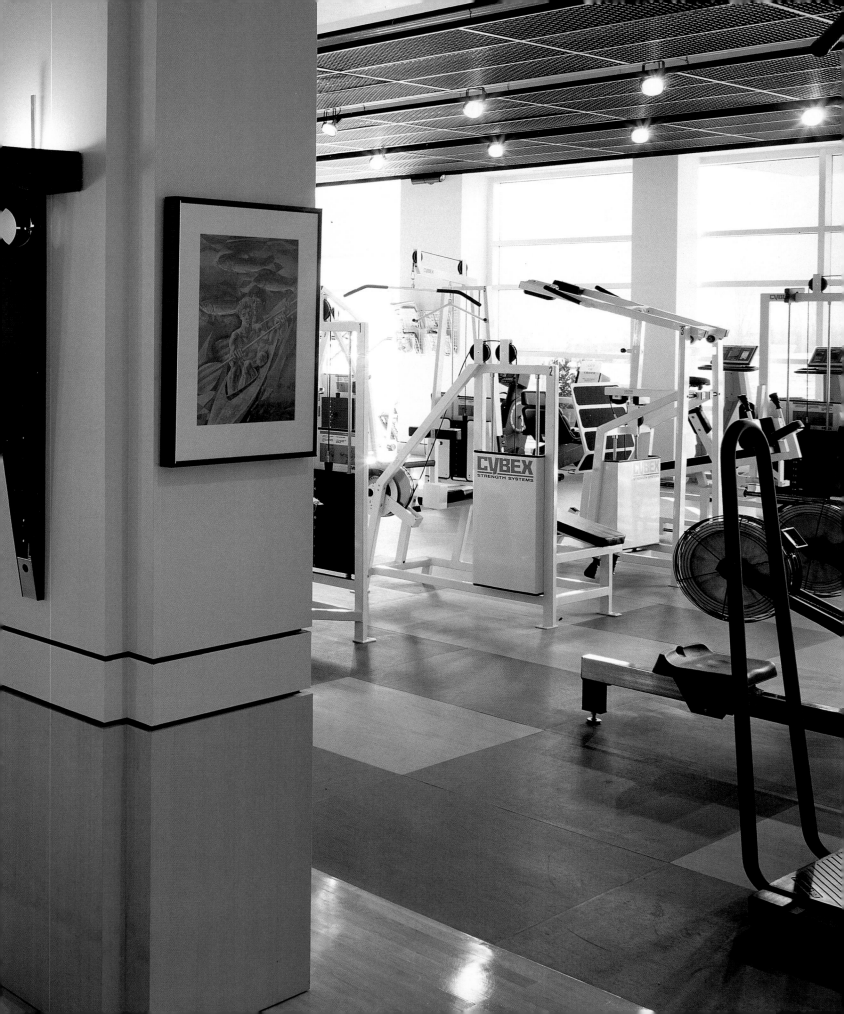

More members and more options create a kinetic mix: pools and outdoor facilities, wellness centers or spas, family-friendly spaces. These clubs often anchor a neighborhood or a workplace as a new social venue.

DIVERSI
ENVIRO

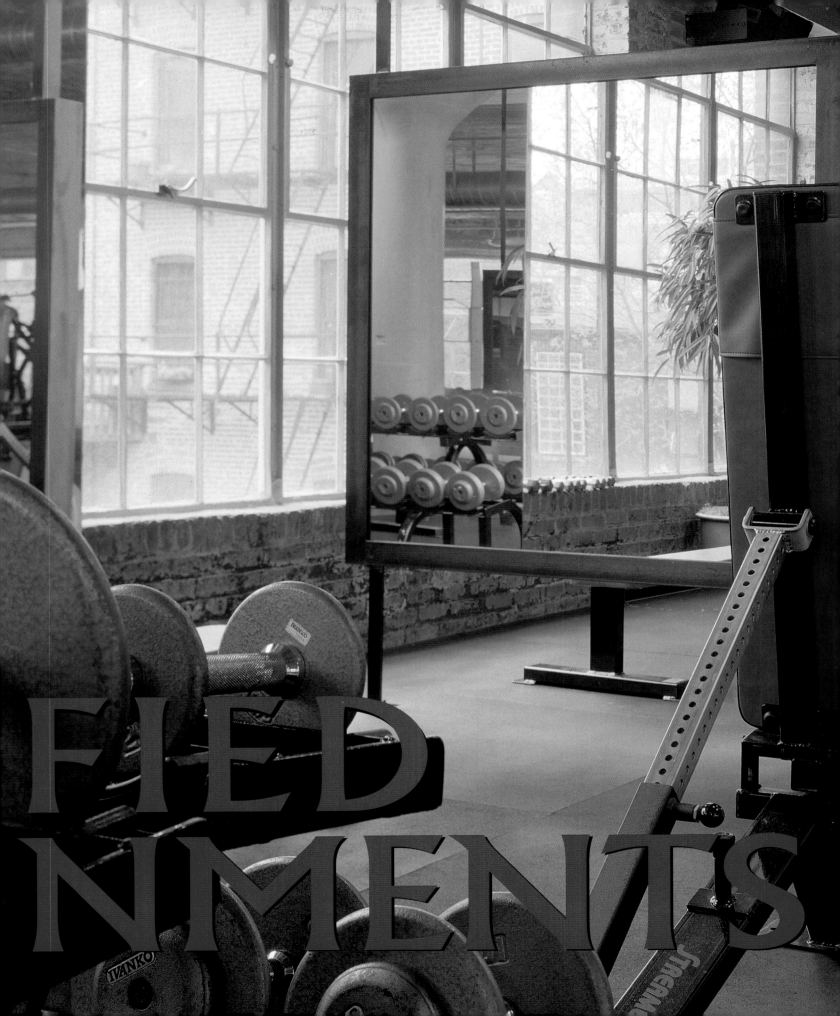

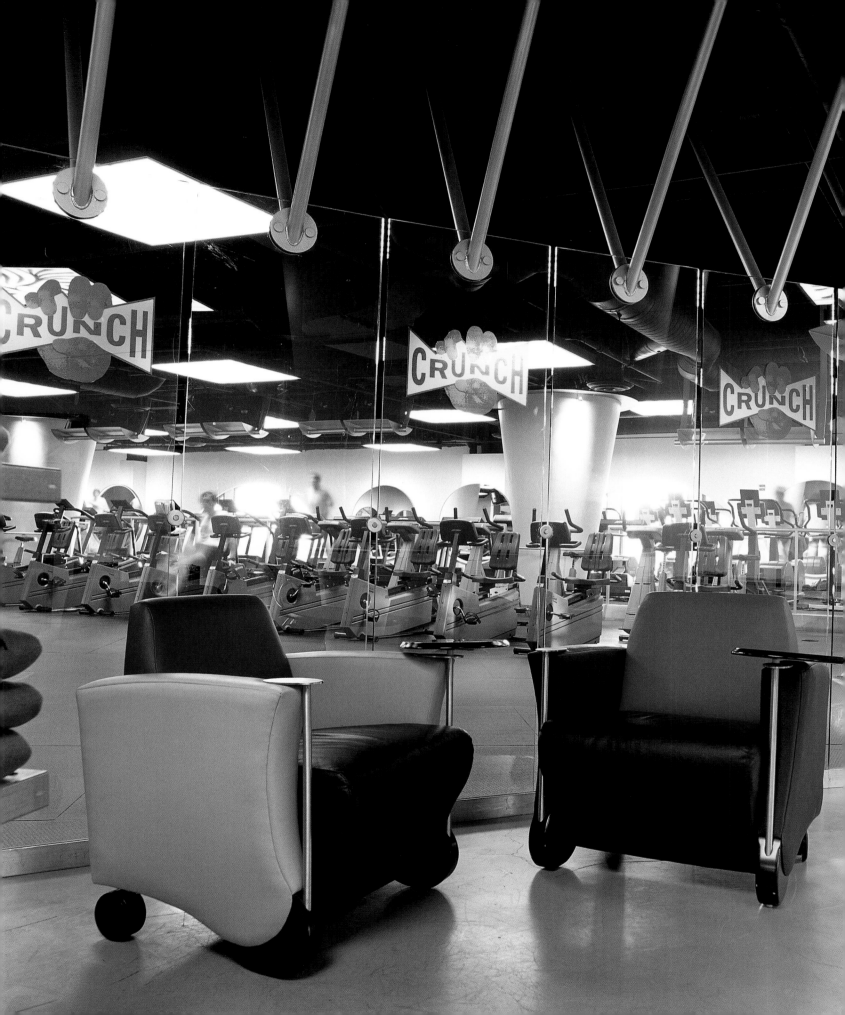

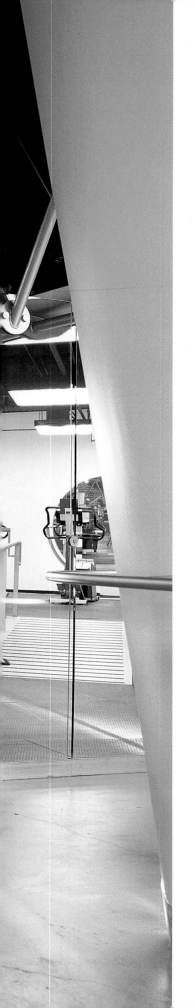

A rchitect Frank Denner has employed the same philosophy to great success, for all six health clubs he's designed for Crunch: "I draw inspiration from the immediate environment to create an original vocabulary with which to build," he says. Indeed, each club captures the spirit of its individual site and surroundings.

The Los Angeles location reflects its setting, offering bright, upbeat, no-frills interiors. Two floors of windows, clear partitions adjacent to workout spaces, and frosted-glass showers fronting the locker-room

hallway create a communal, open atmosphere. The architect employed industrial materials such as stainless steel, glass, and wood juxtaposed with wall murals and swaths of yellow and red (Crunch's signature colors).

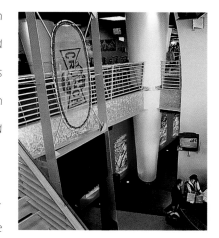

For the New York City location, the sunlight and transparency of the Los Angeles club is replaced with a nightclub mood. The result is a raw space with quirky retail, lighting, and custom-designed locker room fixtures. Exposed brick walls, skylights, and pared-down materials like granite, steel, and wood are countered by inspirational murals and accents of yellow and red. A custom granite-topped reception desk and metal colonnade smoothly direct visitors toward an awkwardly located stairway. The four-story club features cardiovascular and strength training equipment, boxing, spinning, aerobics, and a lounge and juice bar. Crunch has three additional New York City locations and clubs in San Francisco and Tokyo.

CRUNCH

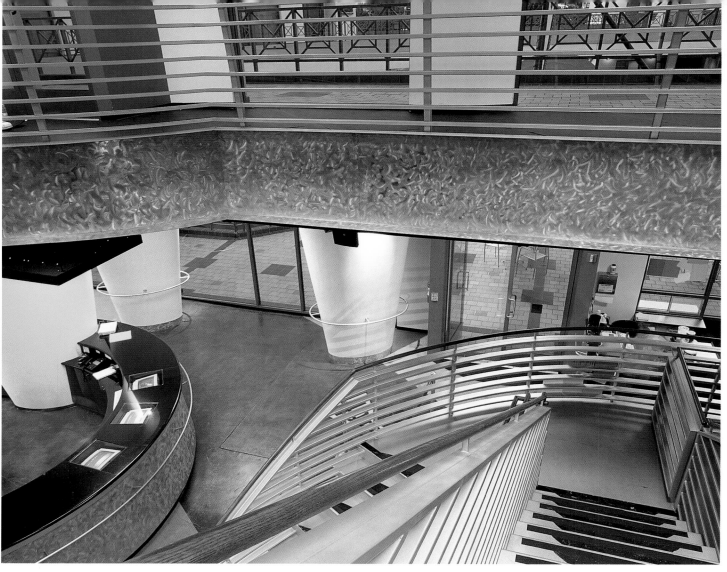

Los Angeles

PREVIOUS SPREAD The lounge area captures the club's energy through clear partitions to the workout space. ABOVE The double-height lobby has pared-down materials and an open plan. BELOW The signature red and yellow dorsal-fin Crunch sign is eye-catching even on busy Sunset Boulevard. OPPOSITE Alluring frosted glass showers bring the locker-room hallway to life.

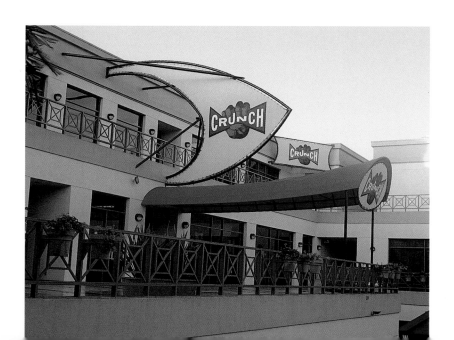

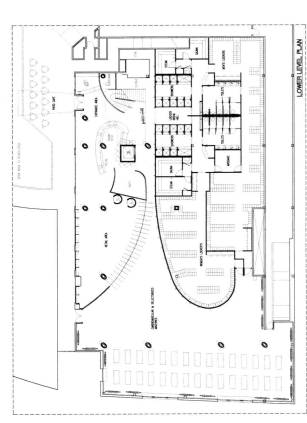

LOWER LEVEL PLAN

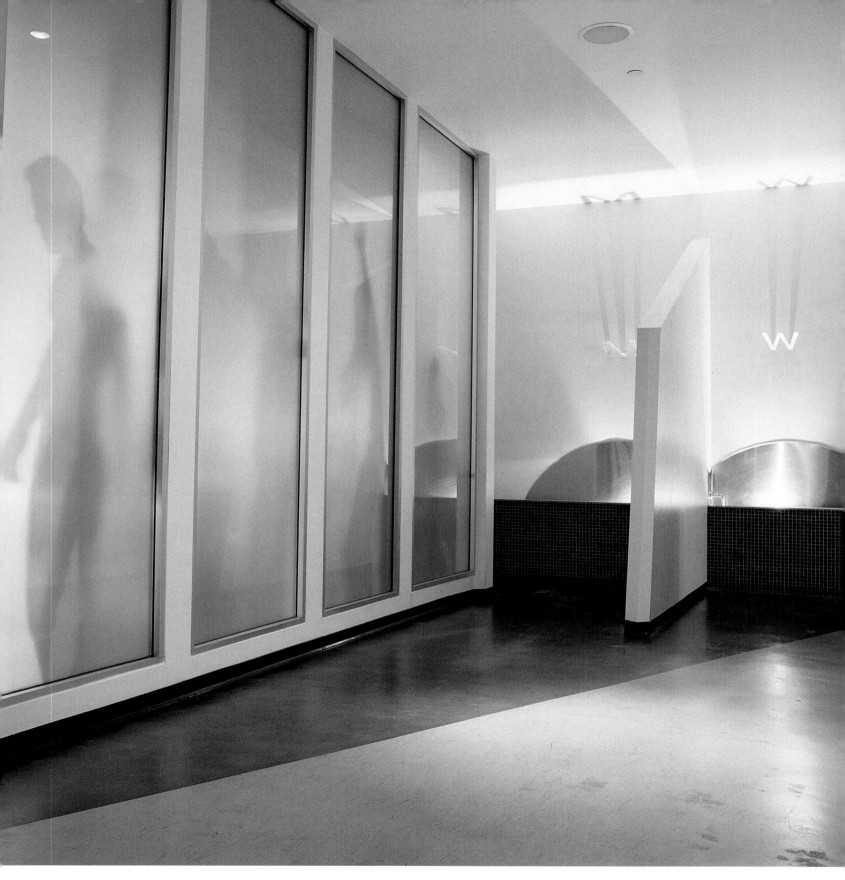

location: **Los Angeles, California**
architects: **Frank Denner Architect; Gensler**
interior designer: **Frank Denner Architect**
photographer: **E.J. Camp**
square feet/meters: **28,000/2,601**
design budget: **$1.4 million**

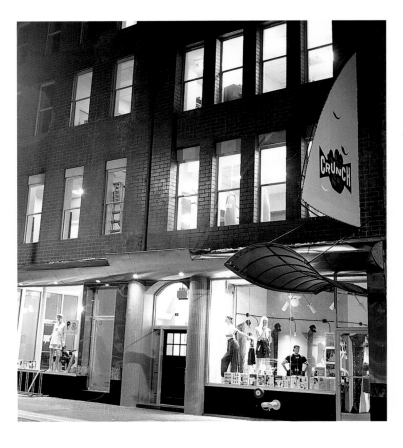

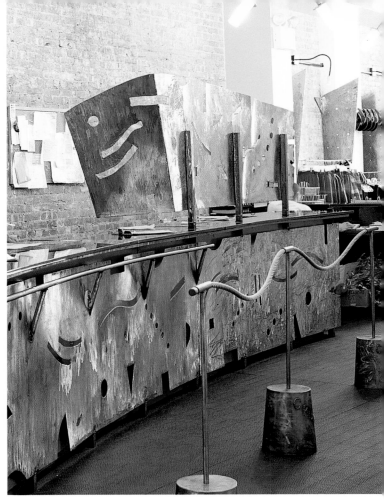

New York

ABOVE Designed with plate-glass windows and dramatic lighting, the club maintains an inviting presence at night. **ABOVE RIGHT** A custom-designed reception desk, handrail, and metal framework help guide visitors to the awkwardly sited stairway. **BELOW RIGHT** Denner's unique split light fixtures highlight the quirky retail space at the front of the gym. **BELOW** The boxing area displays the signature red and yellow Crunch colors. **OPPOSITE ABOVE & CENTER** Exposed-brick walls and industrial-style piping lend urban chic to the cardiovascular and strength training areas. **OPPOSITE BELOW** Rich mahogany is punctuated by leopard-print upholstery in this seating area.

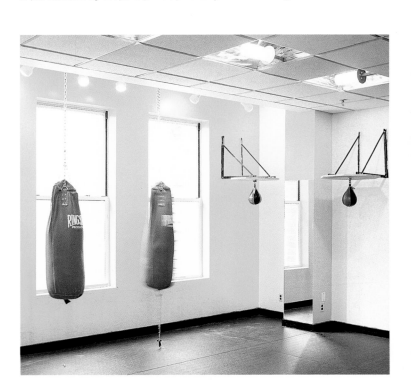

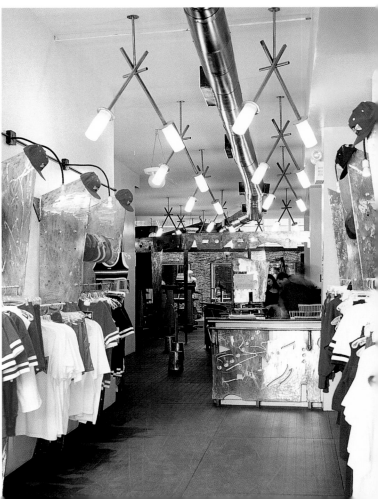

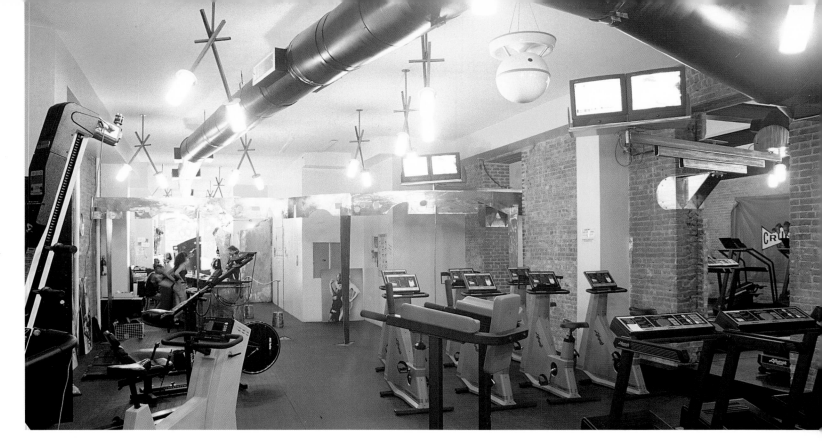

location: **New York, New York**
architect/interior designer: **Frank Denner Architect**
photographer: **Joseph Sinnott**
square feet/meters: **16,000/1,486**
design budget: **$200,000**
club membership: **4,000**

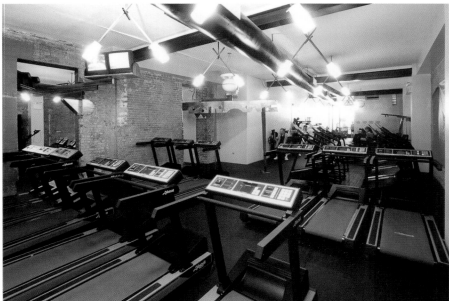

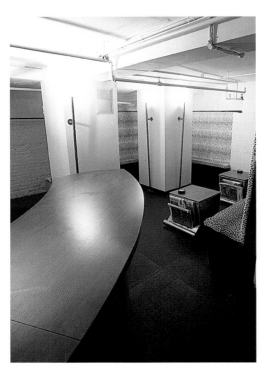

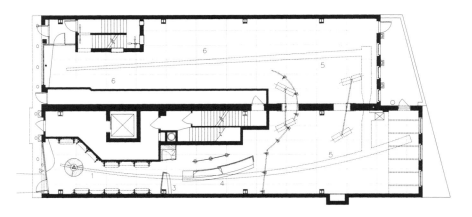

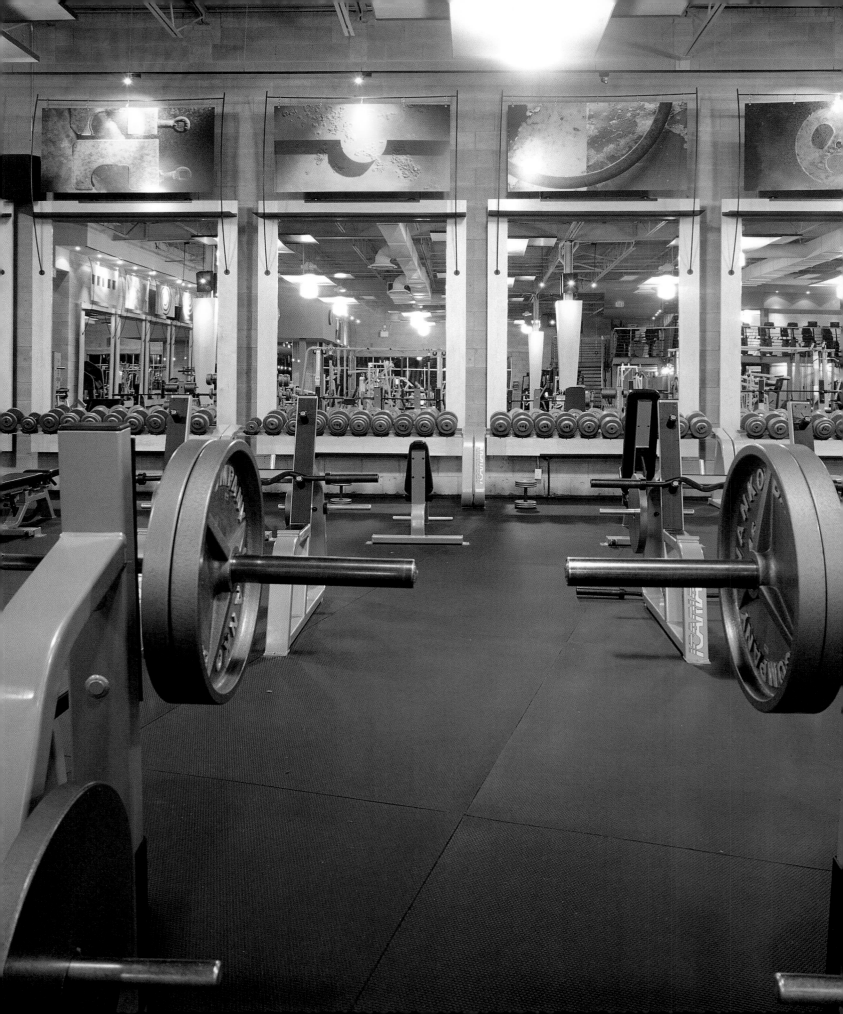

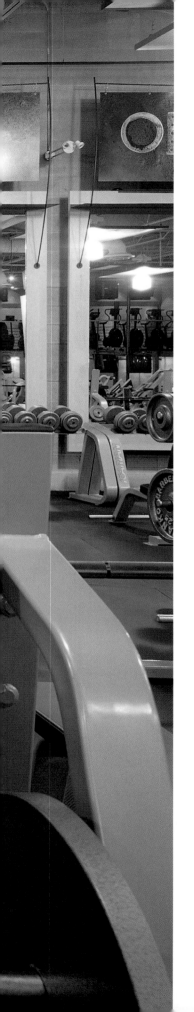

The owners of Ontario's Extreme Fitness are firm believers in the power of good design. Based solely on II BY IV Design Associates' presentation boards and sketches for their planned health club, they were able to sell four thousand advance memberships, financing its construction. And the club has lived up to its buzz, offering a welcoming, state-of-the-art, safe atmosphere for both families and young professionals.

To make a vast abandoned warehouse more intimate in scale, the designers created discrete pockets of space with an overall design coherence—no easy task since the pool, chiropractic, and other services are operated by separate companies that lease the space. Walls punctured with large industrial-style windows provide light and views, and accent lighting flatters both patrons and the architecture. Warm earth tones of ocher, gray, cream, and tan soften industrial materials like masonite,

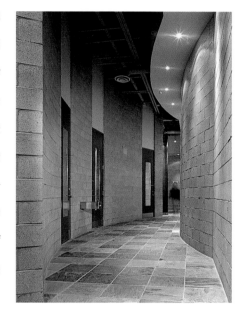

metal, slate, and concrete block, while wood detailing and numerous photographs offer visual interest. Full-height mirrors, individually lit vanities, and private showers provide human-scale comfort. Locker rooms are designed for boys and girls, as well as children's fitness areas. Other features include an elevated indoor track, massage, aerobics, aquatics, a pro shop and juice bar.

EXTREME FITNESS

location: **Thornhill, Ontario**
architect/interior designer: **II BY IV Design Associates Inc.**
photographer: **David Whittaker**
square feet/meters: **27,000/2,508**
design budget: **$850,000**
club membership: **4,000**

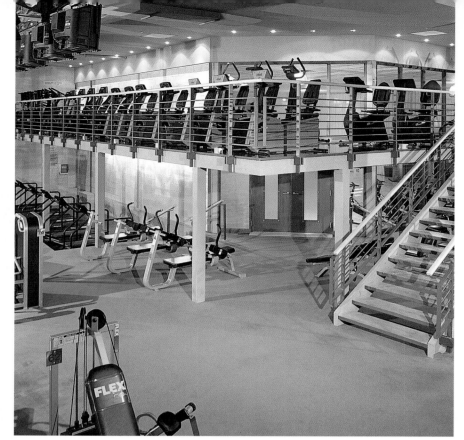

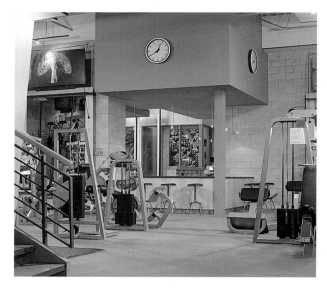

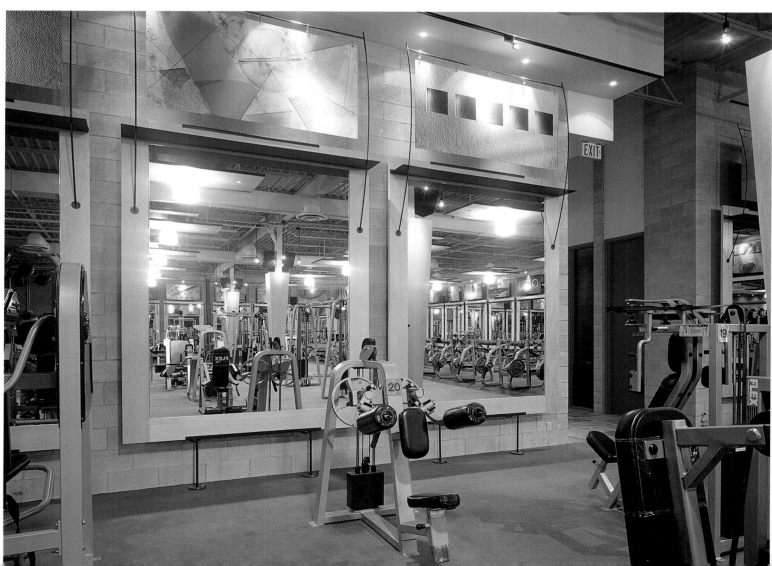

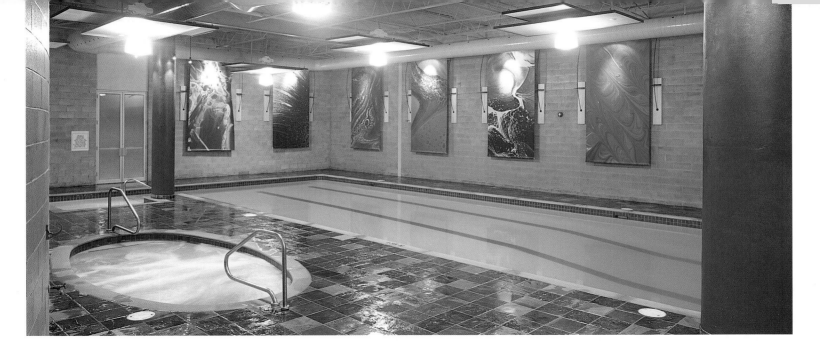

PREVIOUS SPREAD & OPPOSITE BELOW Indirect wall washers highlight the texture of the concrete block, while adding color and softening the materials. Individual full-height mirrors instead of mirrored walls in the weight training area lend a more human scale. OPPOSITE ABOVE LEFT A juice bar located on the weights floor creates an atmosphere for relaxing as well as training. OPPOSITE ABOVE RIGHT The double-height cardiovascular area makes the most of the lofty former warehouse, with a mezzanine level and enclosed aerobics studio. ABOVE The use of bold photography in the pool area and throughout offers interest and polish. RIGHT The designers downsized the vast warehouse with discrete pockets of space, even in the changing rooms, to make them seem more welcoming. All vanities have individual lighting. BELOW RIGHT The spacious juice bar creates a venue for socializing for families and single patrons alike.

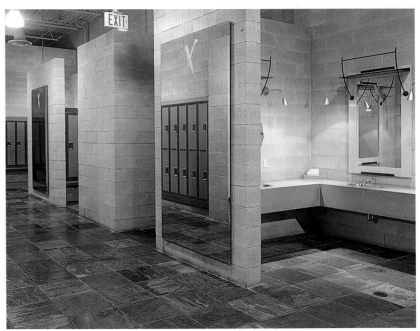

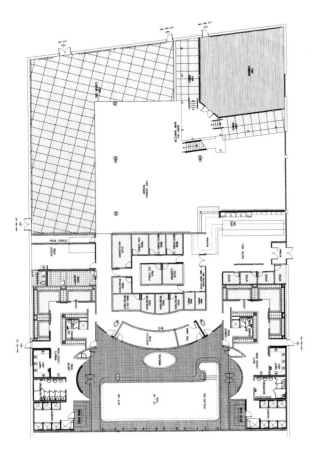

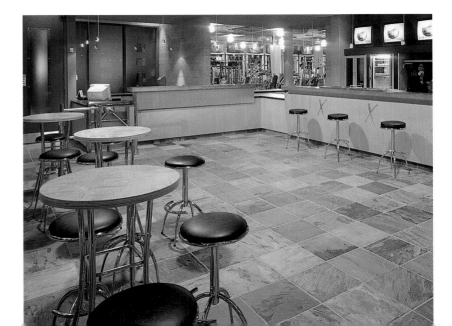

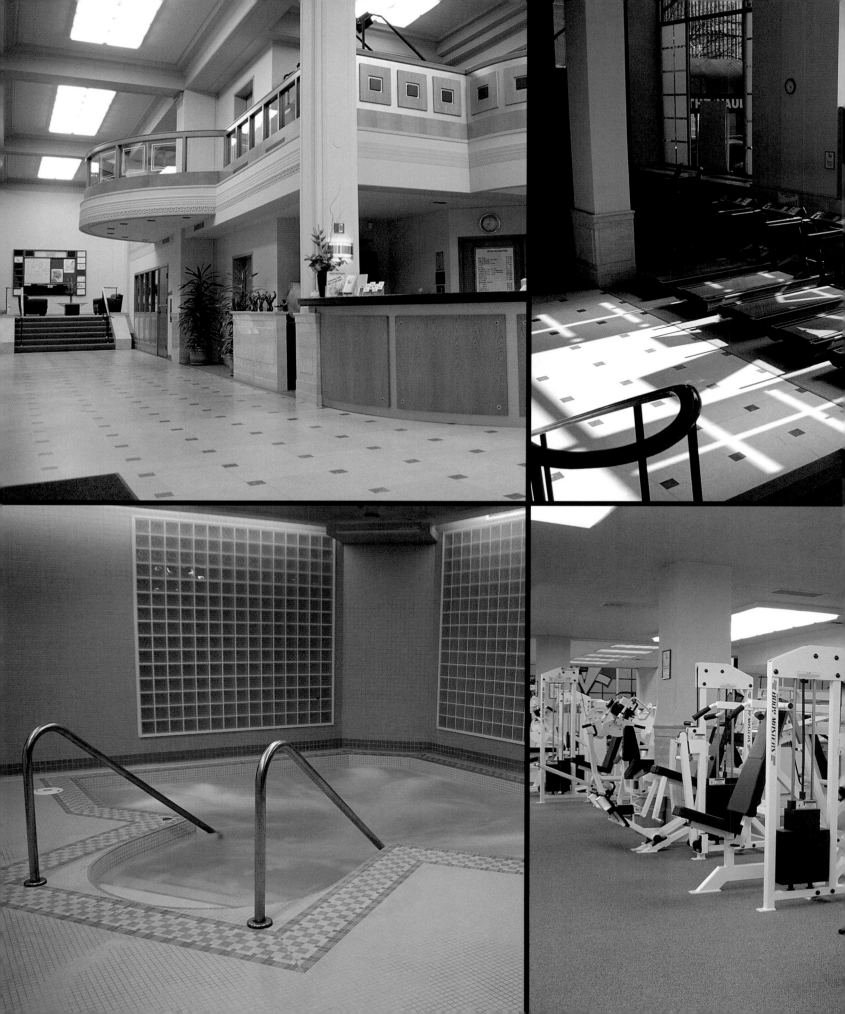

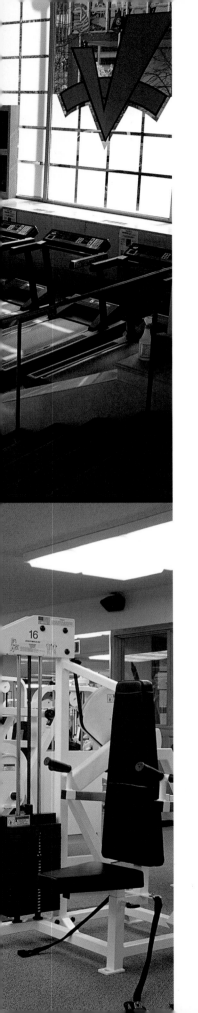

The convenient location, high ceilings, and good bones of a turn-of-the-century bank proved to be the perfect setting for the Vault Fitness Club, a new health club in downtown Seattle. What better place to make the neighborhood professionals feel at ease? As designed by Olympic Associates and Siso Design, the unique details and stately spaces of the 33,000-square-foot landmark building have been given an entirely new context.

The first sign of transformation is evident in the lobby where the old teller counter has become a grand reception desk, with curved, elegant wood paneling that tempers the room's rectilinear form. On the first floor, the bank's massive windows admit natural light to exercisers on the treadmills and circuit training equipment, but the panes are strategically frosted to temper the light and offer privacy. The mezzanine houses

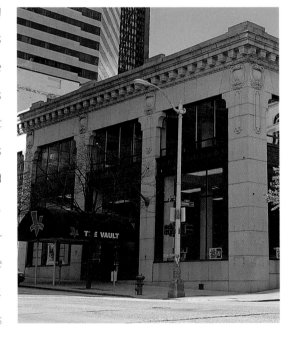

cardiovascular equipment and TV monitors under skylit ceilings. The former vault is announced by a ten-foot waterfall; behind the original door, a coed Jacuzzi is cached. The Vault also features childcare, aerobics, yoga, massage, and spinning facilities, as well as steam rooms, dry saunas and tanning rooms.

THE VAULT FITNESS CLUB

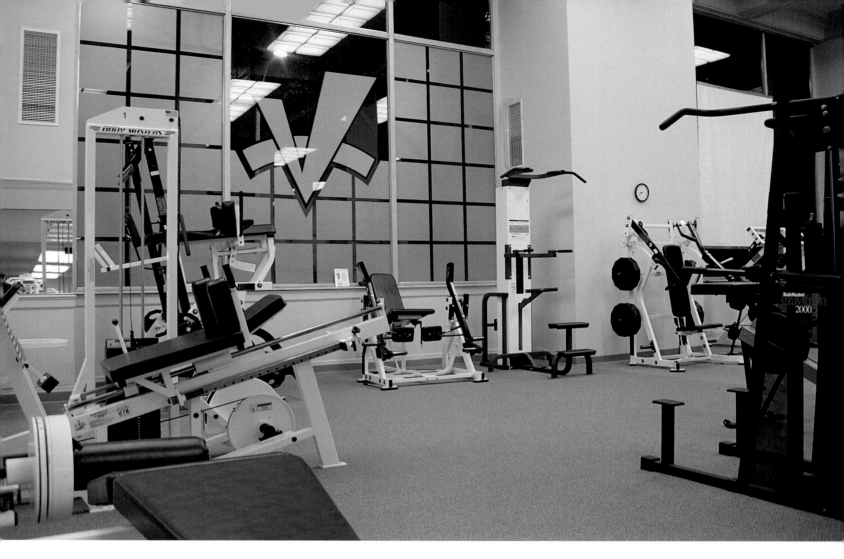

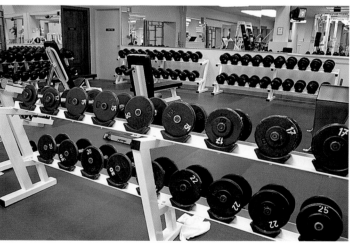

location: Seattle, Washington
architect: Olympic Associates
interior designer: Siso Design
photographer: Benham
square feet/meters: 33,000/3066
design budget: not disclosed
club membership: 3,000

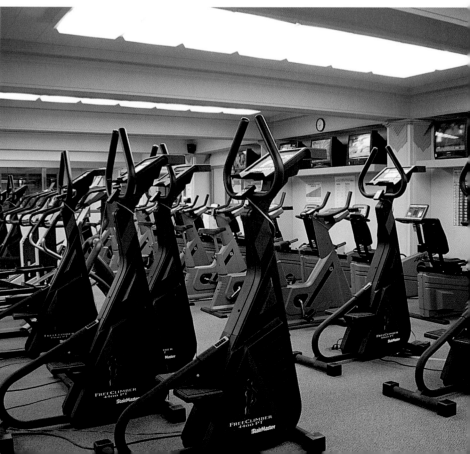

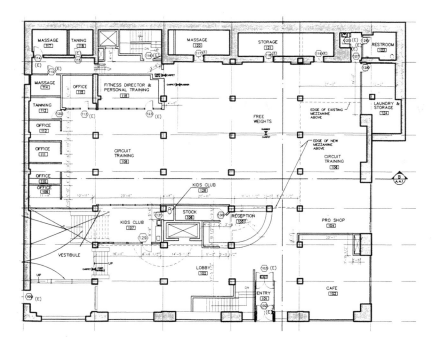

PREVIOUS SPREAD The lobby of the former bank serves as a bright, welcoming gym reception area. Wood paneling, mirrored walls and frosted windows add visual punch to the stately interiors. Glass block windows facing the Jacuzzi create a semiprivate atmosphere for relaxation. OPPOSITE ABOVE The turn-of-the-century building's extra-high ceilings create a comfortable spaciousness in the circuit training area. OPPOSITE BELOW The bank's mezzanine houses much of the cardiovascular equipment, and overlooks the lobby area on one side and television monitors on the other. BELOW The former vault now houses a coed Jacuzzi.

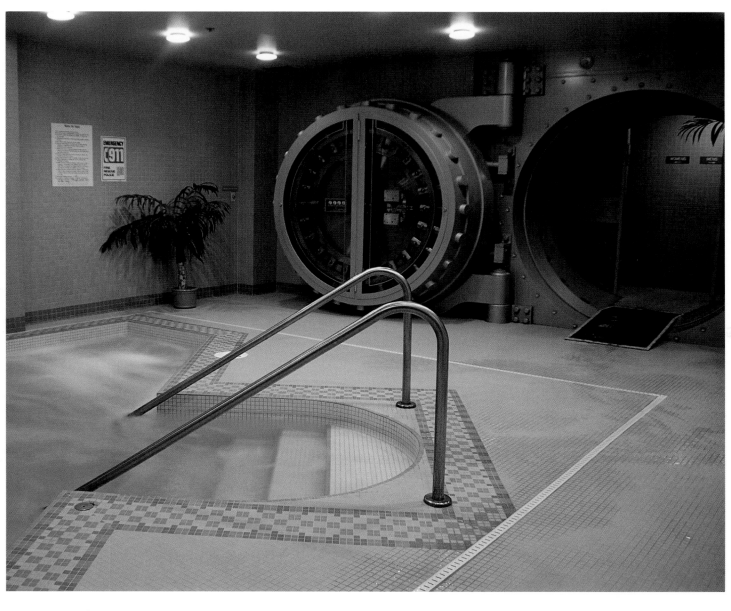

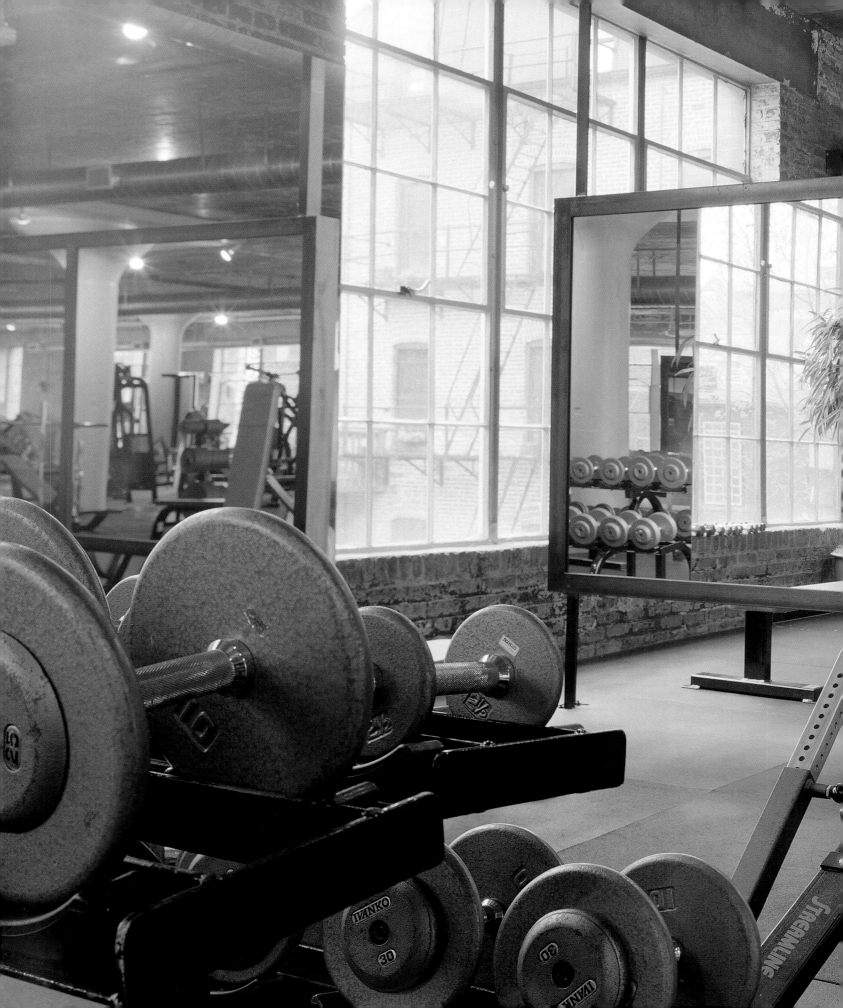

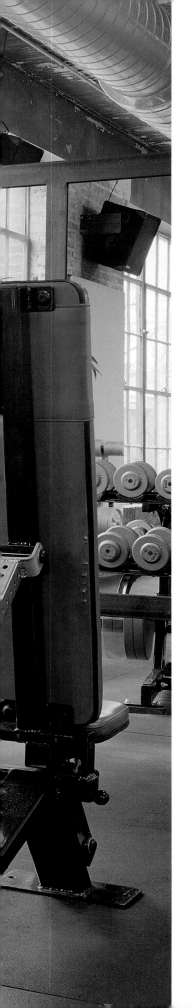

In the diverse Washington, D.C. neighborhood of Adams Morgan, Stoneking/von Storch Architects and club owner Doug Jefferies created a hip, light-filled fitness center that stays true to its industrial roots. "The key to the design's success—as with physical fitness—was not expensive materials," says Michael Stoneking, "but a commitment to the process."

To meet Results' programmatic and technological requirements while preserving the building's architectural integrity, the designers worked with local historic committees on exterior finishes and a new storefront. Inside, steel sash windows were restored and the original brick walls and concrete ceilings left unfinished. The designers located the women's locker room, aerobics studios, and fitness area on the third floor; main cardio-

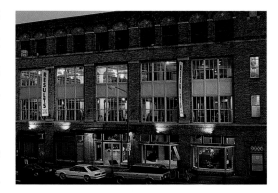

vascular and weight-training area on the second floor; and the men's locker room on the first floor. Tanning, testing, and massage rooms occupy blocky cabanas along the entry corridor.

Combining inexpensive materials, finishes, and lighting to create strong visual and spatial effects, the designers laid out the workout spaces along an existing grid of concrete columns, painted bright yellow. Custom mirrored partitions create more intimate spaces within the overall open plan, and adjustable mirrors mounted on the columns allow members to check their weightlifting technique from any angle.

RESULTS THE GYM

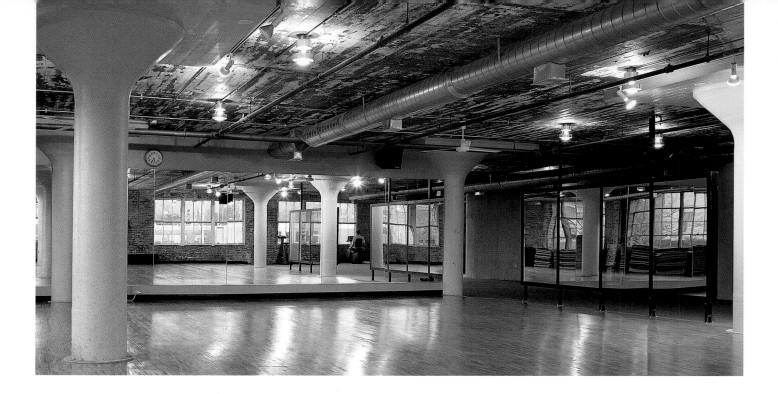

PREVIOUS SPREAD The open free weight area is divided into more intimate spaces with custom-built mirrored partitions. ABOVE & OPPOSITE The weight training and aerobics areas are laid out on an existing grid of large scale concrete columns, painted an eye-catching bright yellow. RIGHT The men's locker room, signaled by a glass block partition and tomato-red wall, reflects Results' modern yet industrial aesthetic.

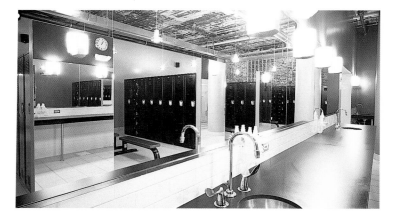

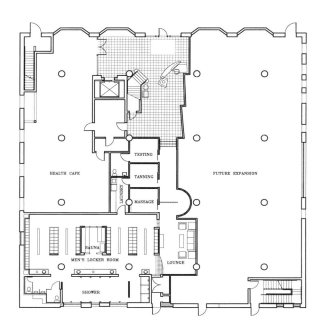

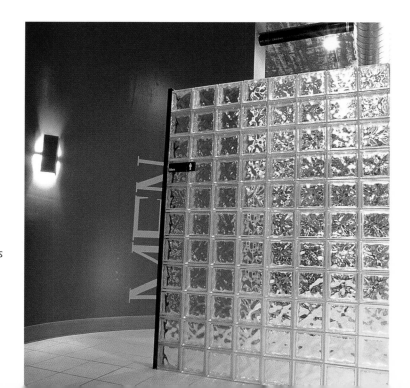

location: Washington, D.C.
architect/interior designer: Stoneking/von Storch Architects
photographer: James Watts
square feet/meters: 25,000/2,323
design budget: $590,000
club membership: 1,800

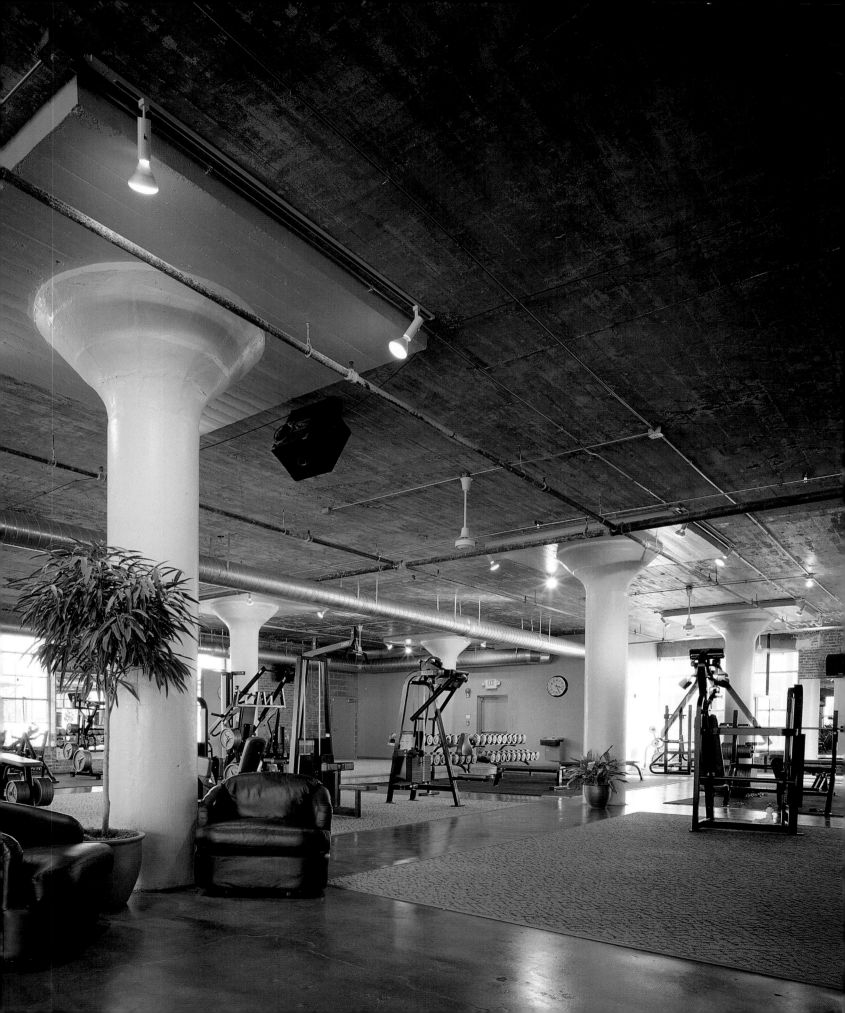

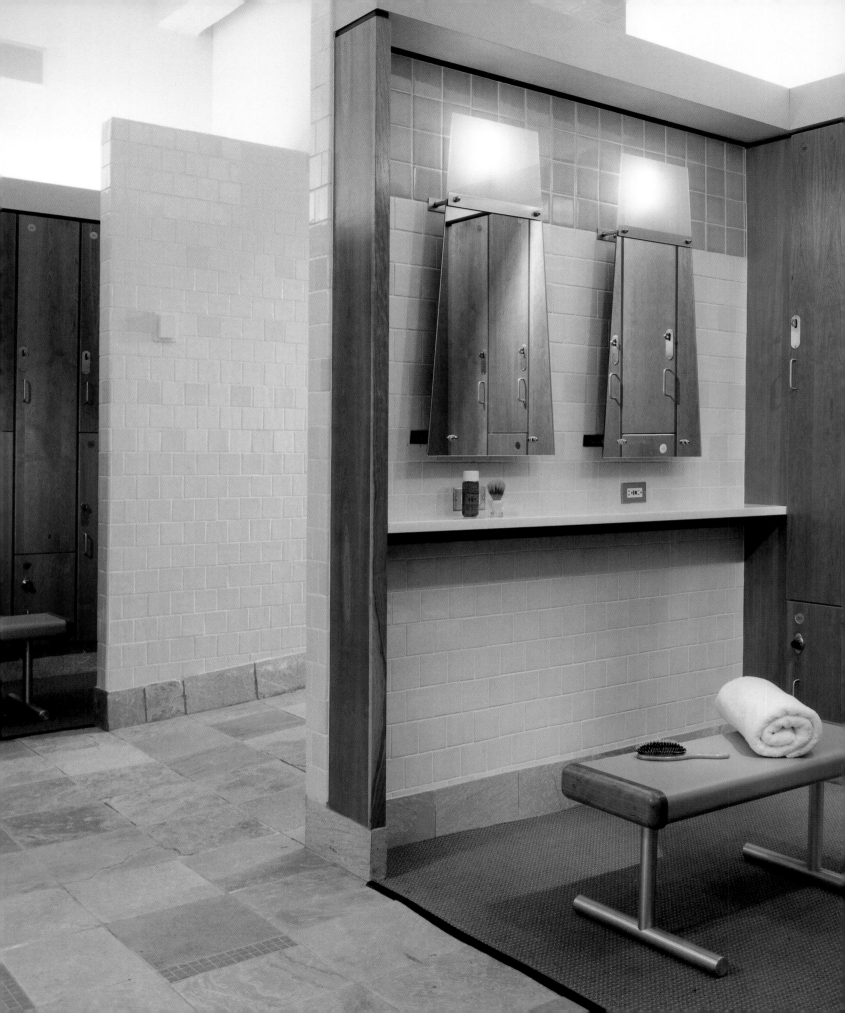

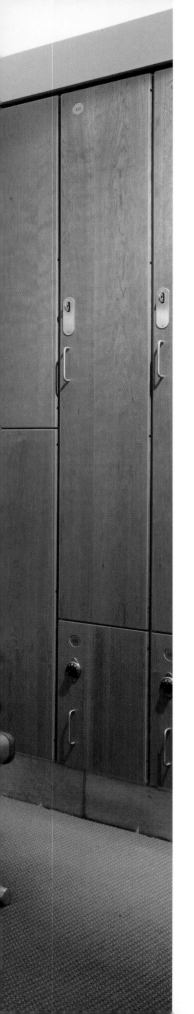

H LW International assisted Equinox Fitness Clubs in elevating their concept to the next level: integrating an exercise facility with a full-service Equinox Urban Spa/Clarins Institute, food and retail spaces, and nutrition center to create a four-story shrine to health and well-being. Equinox's Upper East Side location is targeted to its "upper-mass-market neighborhood, with a focus on great services, products, and environments," says HLW's Paul Boardman. The club promotes a kinder, gentler workout, injecting light, openness, and air into the urban-chic ethic.

The entry recalls a luxury hotel, with a sweeping canopy of perforated metal and glass, custom torchieres, and a first-floor concierge desk. The palette of high-end materials like Brazilian quartzite, cast glass,

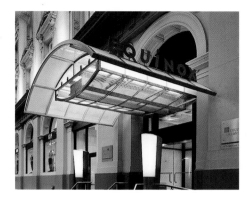

cherry wood, and handcrafted finishes is established here. The second floor is awash with natural light from oversized windows, with sculptural white sailcloth shades tempering the brightness. The spa is cached in a serene, gift-wrapped suite of rooms—the physical and thematic center of the gym. A cocoon of cherry walls and acoustical privacy adds to the calm. Up the central staircase are the two exercise floors, where the mood intensifies: celadon and off-white colors are replaced with jewel tones. The aerobics studio has a generous skylit roof, and equipment is sited along the windows to treat the majority of New Yorkers who don't have a view. The locker rooms are an exerciser's delight, with wood lockers, ivory walls, and plenty of space for space's sake.

EQUINOX FITNESS CLUBS

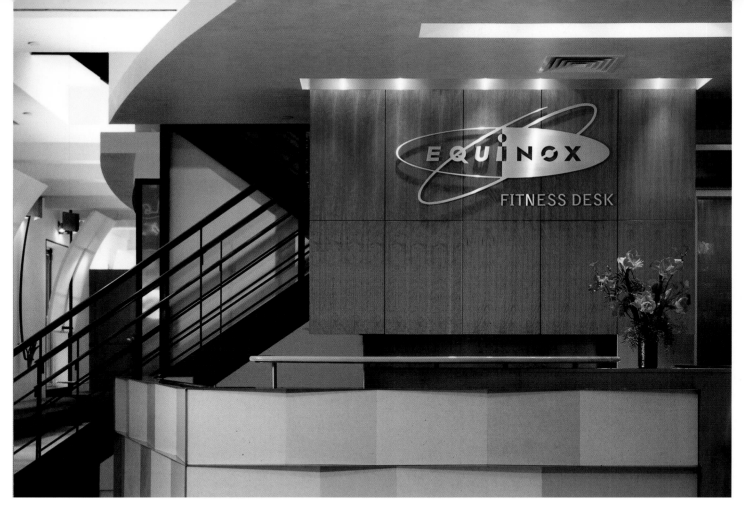

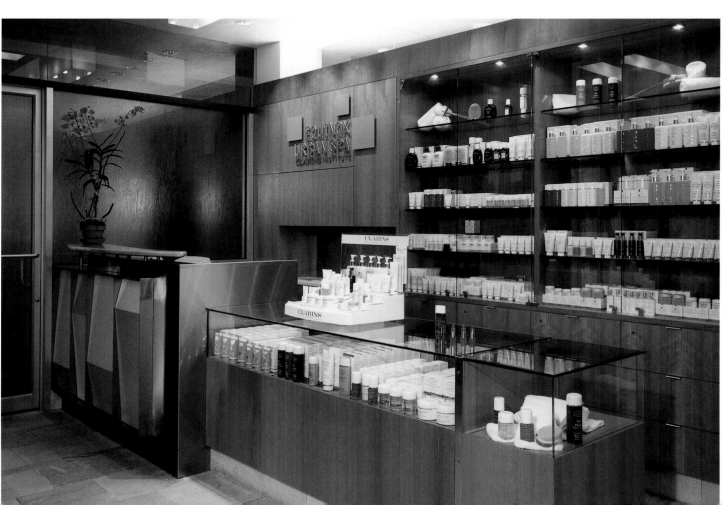

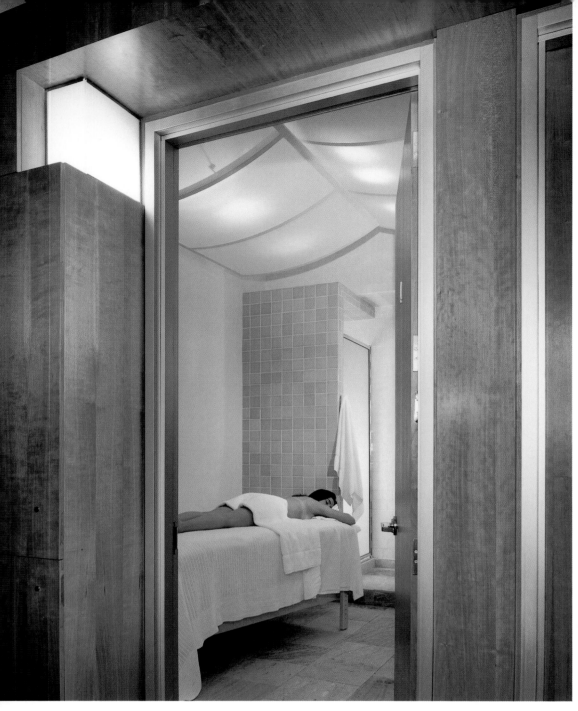

PREVIOUS SPREAD Locker rooms are delightfully spacious with wood lockers, custom light fixtures and distinctive mirrors. An eye-catching exterior canopy and torchieres attract members to the club entrance. The canopy establishes the intimate, service-oriented hotel aesthetic. OPPOSITE ABOVE The first-floor reception area establishes the materials palette and spa hues of celadon and ivory. OPPOSITE BELOW A retail area featuring Clarins products is finished in cherry wood and brushed stainless steel. LEFT Rooms are cocoon-like spaces, with quartzite floors, pale tile walls, and custom light fixtures.

location: New York, New York
architect/interior designer: HLW International LLP
photographer: Peter Paige
square feet/meters: 40,000/3,720
design budget: $3 million
club membership: 5,000

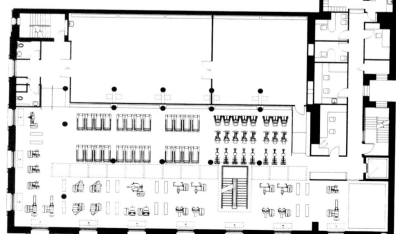

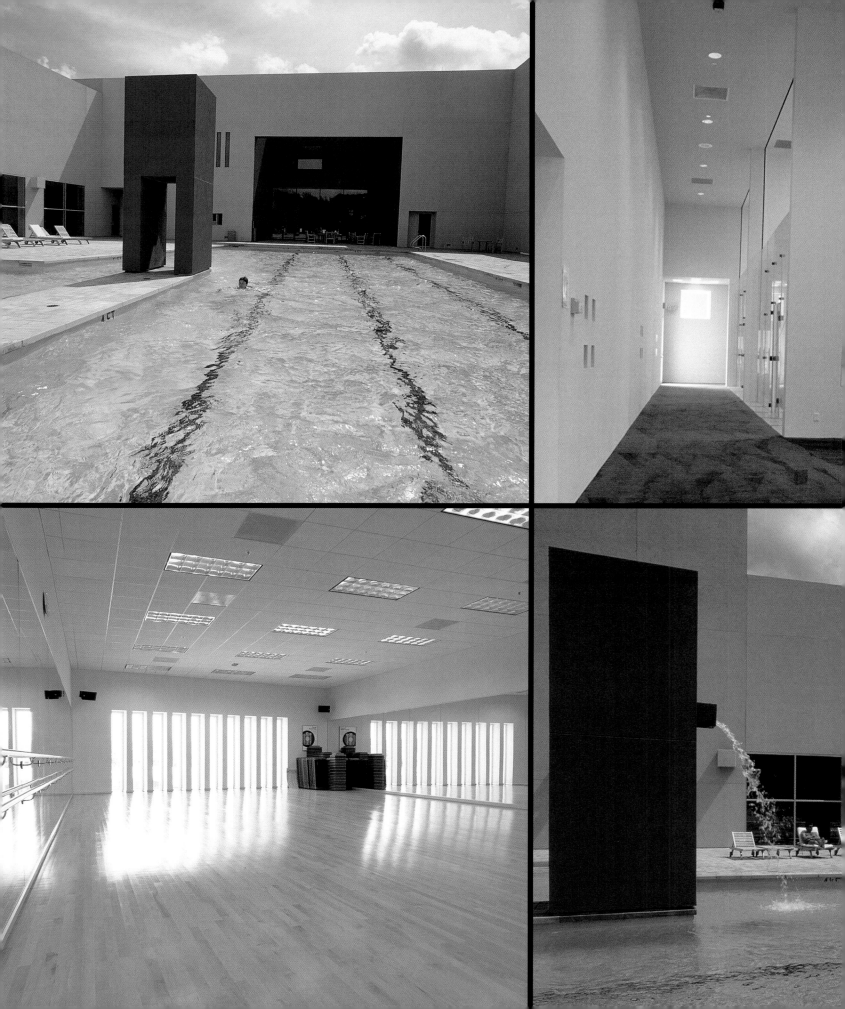

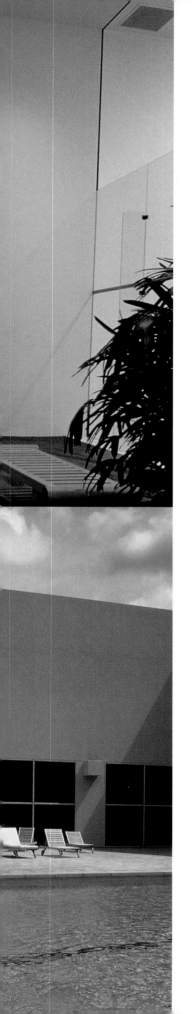

S olana, a 1,600-acre development and office park located outside of Dallas, Texas, avoids the downfalls of most office parks (isolating design, lack of cohesion, few amenities) through a reverential connection to the environment. Landscaping is based on the site's rolling hills, prairies, and native growth, and the structure reflects the architects' regional influences from Mexico. Legorreta Arquitectos was one of several architects who worked on Solana, incorporating IBM's massive complex and the Village Center across the highway, which includes a hotel, two office buildings, restaurants—and a breathtaking sports facility.

The fitness center draws on the architects' overall themes, creating a powerful interplay of simple forms, brilliant colors, and dramatic shadows. A dazzling central outdoor pool refers to the Mexican Colonial-style 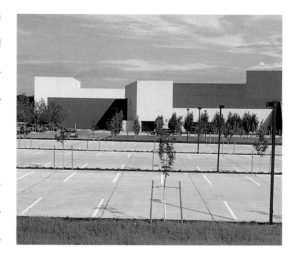 plaza, around which cluster low-rise buildings housing an indoor pool, aerobics studio, dining area, and equipment room. Interiors are flooded with Texas sun dramatized by a diversity of window sizes and shapes. Both indoors and out the architects punctuated spaces with saturated color: inky blue forms and wall faces in the pool plaza, and lacquered floors in the training room create intense environments. The carefully designed spaces humanize the boundless Texas prairie, creating an emotional connection with the land.

THE SOLANA CLUB

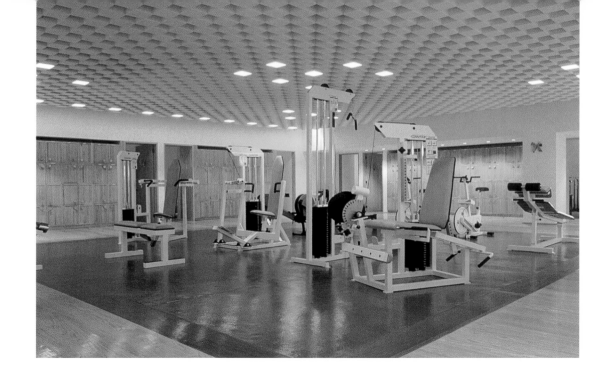

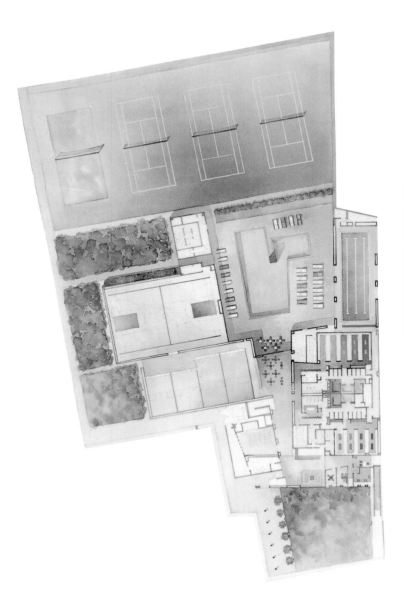

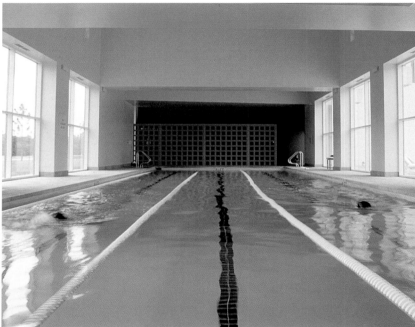

PREVIOUS SPREAD The central outdoor pool illustrates Legorreta's interplay of varying-scale walls, color, and fenestration. Double-height window walls admit light to interior corridors. The aerobics studio is illuminated by windows which are reflected by mirrored walls. TOP A blood-red floor is a single splash of color in the neutral-toned weight-training room. ABOVE An indoor pool overlooks the outdoor one, accented by refreshing swaths of red and blue. OPPOSITE Exterior window patterns are echoed in interior wall partitions in the dining room.

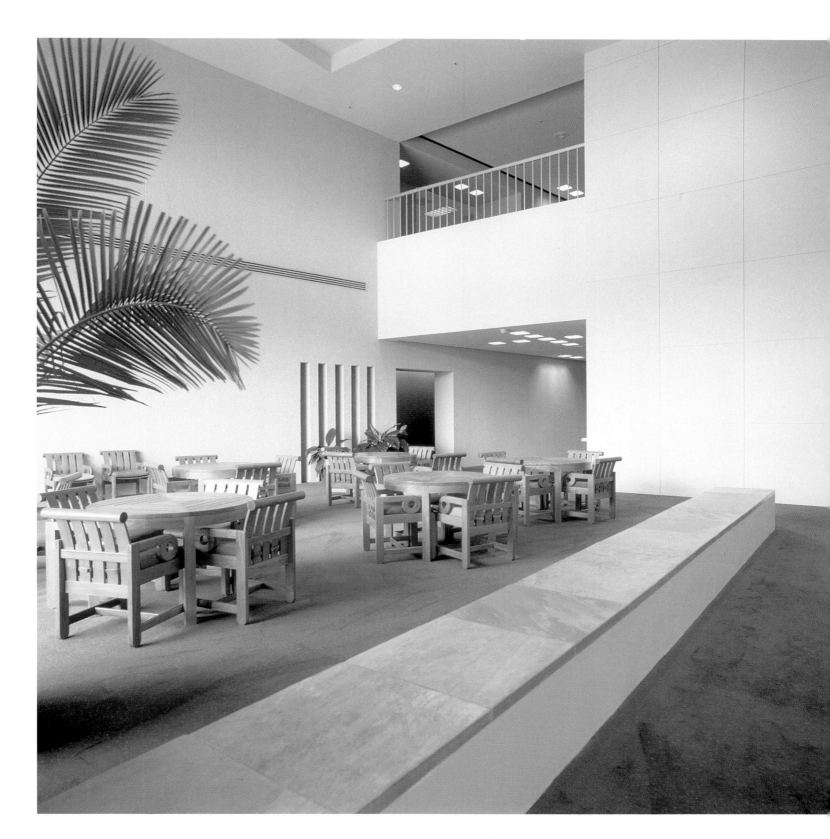

location: **Westlake, Texas**
architect/interior designer: **Legorreta Arquitectos**
photographer: **Lourdes Legorreta**
square feet/meters: **40,000/3,716**
design budget: **not disclosed**
club membership: **3,000**

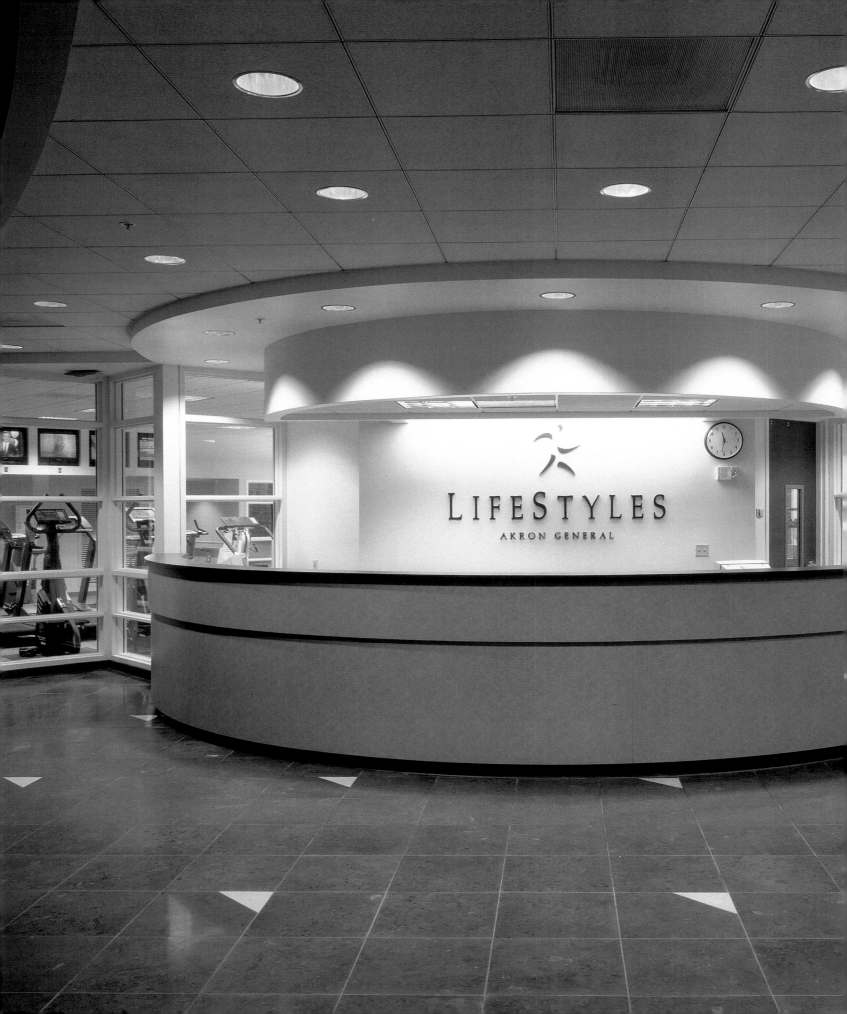

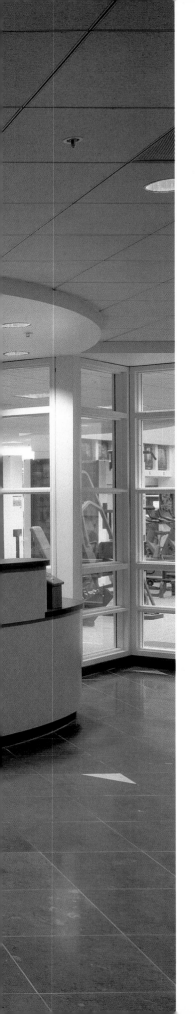

B efore designing the Akron General Health and Wellness Center, The Insights Group interviewed key personnel and visited existing facilities across the country that reflect the evolution of healthcare toward integrating medicine and wellness. The resulting center combines fitness/wellness membership programs, physical therapy, sports medicine, cardiopulmonary rehabilitation, women's health programs, diagnostic services, outpatient surgery, physicians' offices, and conference facilities. The design challenge was to express this integration architecturally.

Upon entering, one feels a sense of well-being and sees people actively involved in getting fit. The extensive use of glass on exterior and interior walls invites views through the exercise floor and the pools beyond. In physical therapy 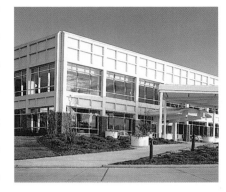 and cardiovascular rehabilitation areas, the floor plan accommodates both private and semiprivate treatment/exams. The absence of walls promotes commingling of therapeutic, clinical and wellness activities. The building's color palette is drawn from nature, as is the choice of materials: limestone floor tile, wood benches, leaf-patterned carpet, plants, and warm-hued wallcovering and paint. Indirect lighting provides a comfortable, glare-free glow. Other services include spa treatments, babysitting, a restaurant, a health resource library, regular community programs, and a children's wellness center. What is not visible is just as impressive: a vast system of medical, mechanical, communications, electrical, and security technology supports the highly specialized spaces.

AKRON GENERAL
HEALTH AND WELLNESS CENTER

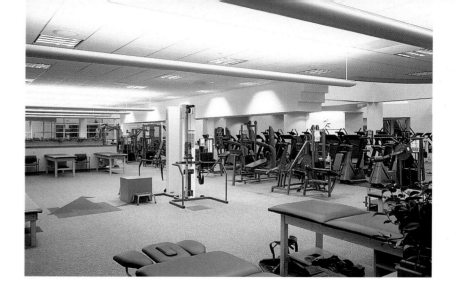

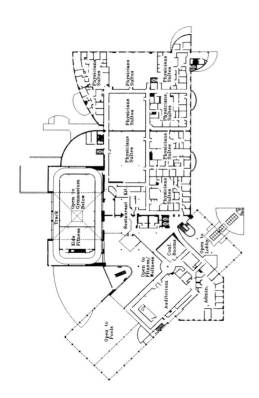

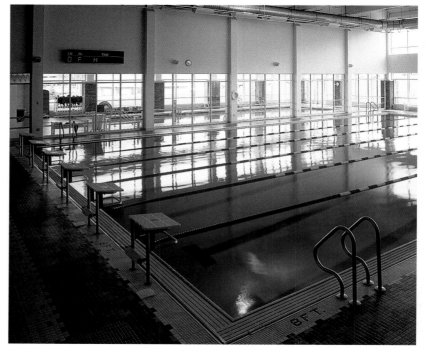

PREVIOUS SPREAD The control desk is surrounded by glass walls, which encourage its use. ABOVE RIGHT The physical therapy area is adjacent to the main exercise floor, promoting patients' speedy recovery. RIGHT Physically separated yet visually connected by a glass wall, the therapy pool and whirlpool areas are finished in warm-colored tile patterns. BELOW RIGHT The children's wellness program is situated on the second floor and is encircled by the indoor running track. BELOW The mezzanine running track overlooks the courts below for visual interest. OPPOSITE Open exercise floors supervised by centrally located desk staff, promote the use of a variety of the club's offerings. Two stories of glass walls bring abundant light to the exercise floors.

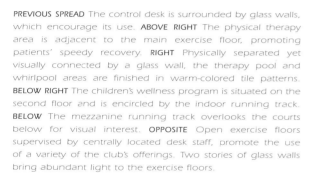

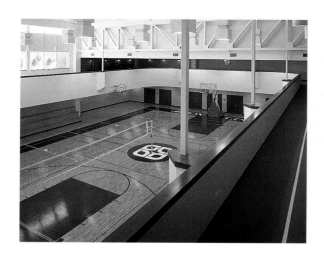

location: **Akron, Ohio**
architect/interior designer: **The Insights Group**
photographer: **Jim Maguire, Akron, Ohio**
square feet/meters: **40,000/3,716**
design budget: **not disclosed**

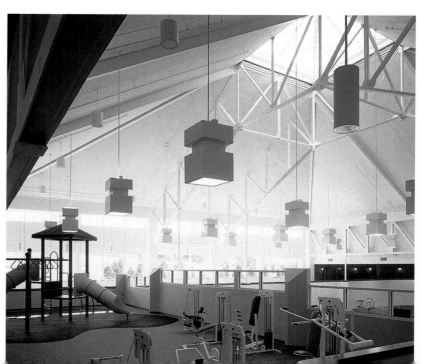

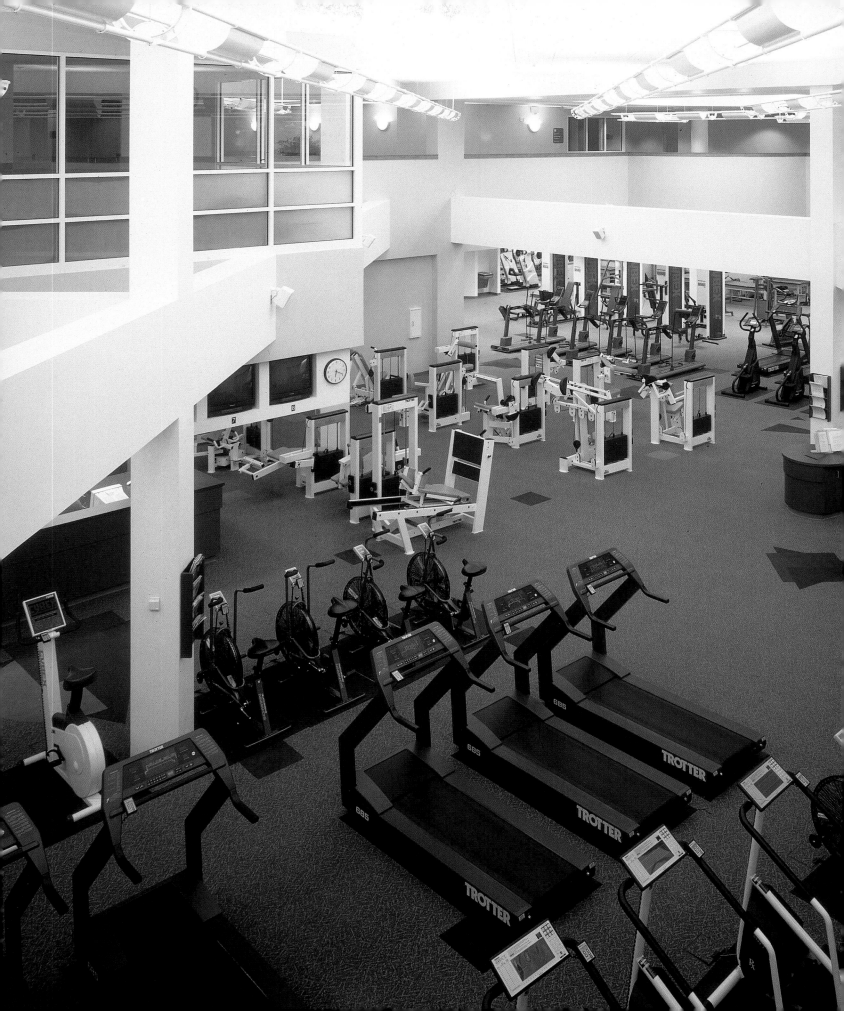

A small, targeted club is often the choice of the professional or city dweller. Service is always at a premium, one-on-one training is the norm, and every square foot demands visual intrigue.

BOUTIQ
GYMS

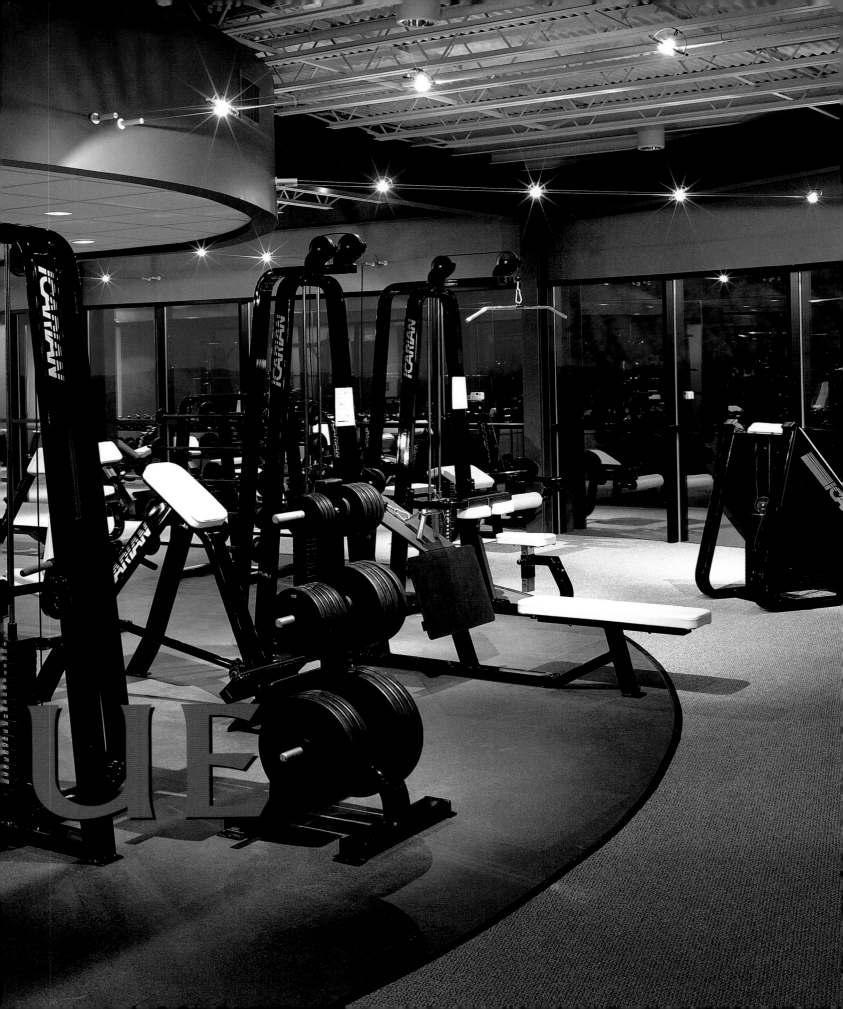

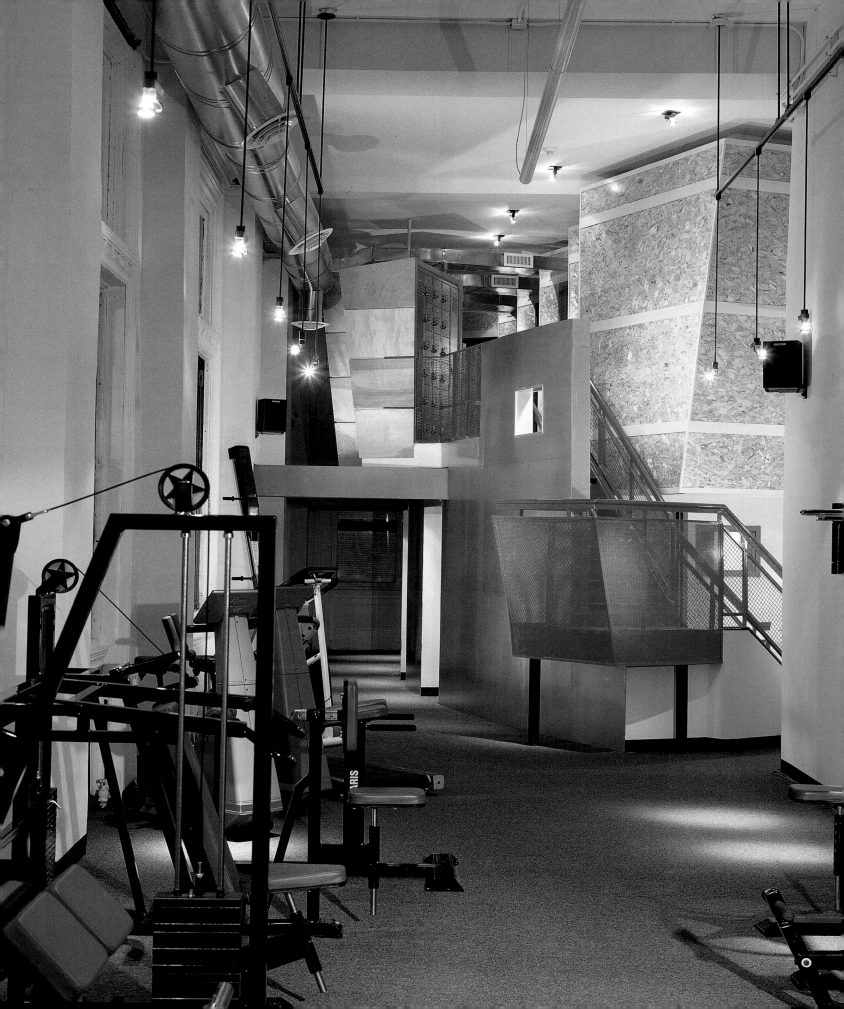

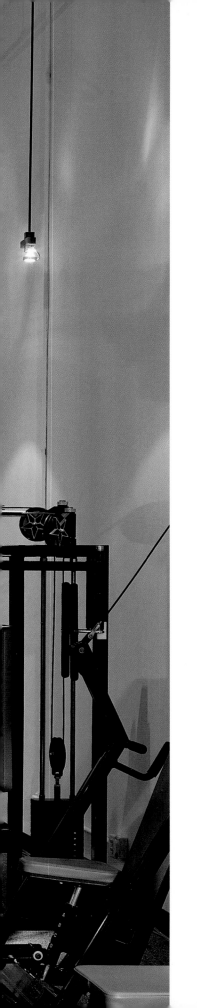

T hanhauser & Esterson Architects' cerebral yet kinetic explorations of health club design began in 1991 with Definitions I, in Manhattan's Wall Street district. The designers' aim was to incite the intense visual movement and shifting perspectives of Deconstructivism, yet preserve a sense of overall form. Combining an existing mezzanine and ground-floor space into a double-height volume, the initial rectilinear plan was compressed to fit the site, causing the walls to curve and fragment, the beams to twist, and ultimately, the locker enclosures and bathroom wall to lean. "It seemed appropriate in a landscape of exercise machines, all designed to orchestrate compressive and tensile forces, that the architecture reflect these forces," says Charles Thanhauser. Welded wire, sheet metal, and aspenite, a wood composite, were selected for their unusual appearance and durability.

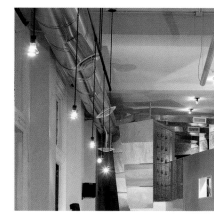

Definitions II, located in a loft in Manhattan's Flatiron district, embodies the tenets of Italian Futurist painting. The designers were intrigued by "voyeurism—real and metaphorical"; the once-overs of one's body and those of others that are a guilty pleasure of gym life. The four shower rooms are enclosed in translucent glass, onto which changers' shadows are cast with bright downlighting. "Having exposed the bodies, it occured to us to expose the architecture," says Thanhauser. Plumbing and electrical lines, ducts, chalk layouts, and plaster patches are left untouched. The interior of Definitions II was exhibited at the

DEFINITIONS FITNESS CENTERS

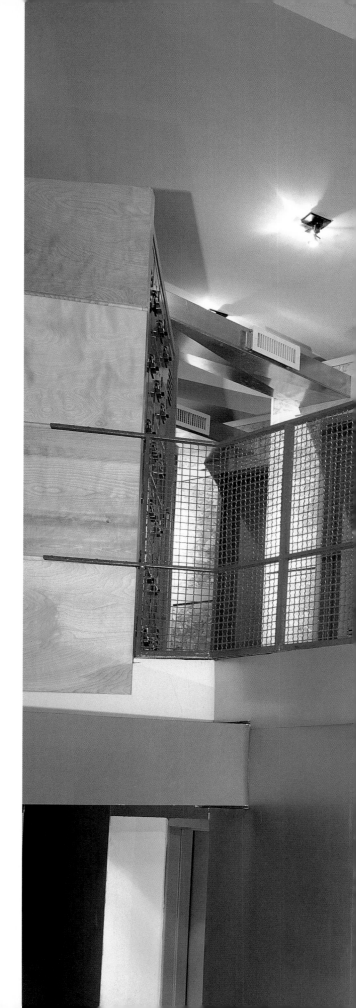

Museum of Modern Art, New York, and the Museu d'Art Contemporani, Barcelona.

For Definitions III, on the upper East Side, a confined area was transformed into a deftly choreographed delight. The site—two apartments joined by a small hallway—did not offer an easy flow of workout spaces. To provide visual movement, the designers manipulated elevations and introduced organic, curvilinear ceiling forms that flow with the plan. The result is a "dramatic contrast to the rectilinear plan," with oblique compositions of the elevations, and wave-like ceiling forms," says Thanhauser. Attention to detail is most evident in lacquered mahogany and maple panels echoed in the changing room wall, and the addition of three types of glass in a steel frame.

location: **New York, New York**
architect/interior designer: **Thanhauser & Esterson Architects P.C.**
photographer: **© Brian Rose**
square feet/meters: **4,000/372**
design budget: **$350,000**

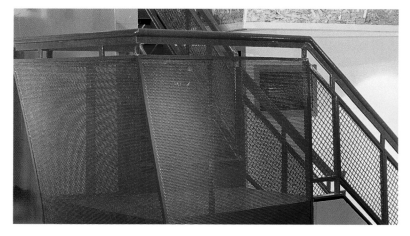

Definitions I

PREVIOUS SPREAD The designers' goal was to incite visual movement and shifting perspectives, yet preserve a sense of overall form. **ABOVE & RIGHT** Materials like welded wire, metal, and aspenite were selected for their unusual appearance and durability.

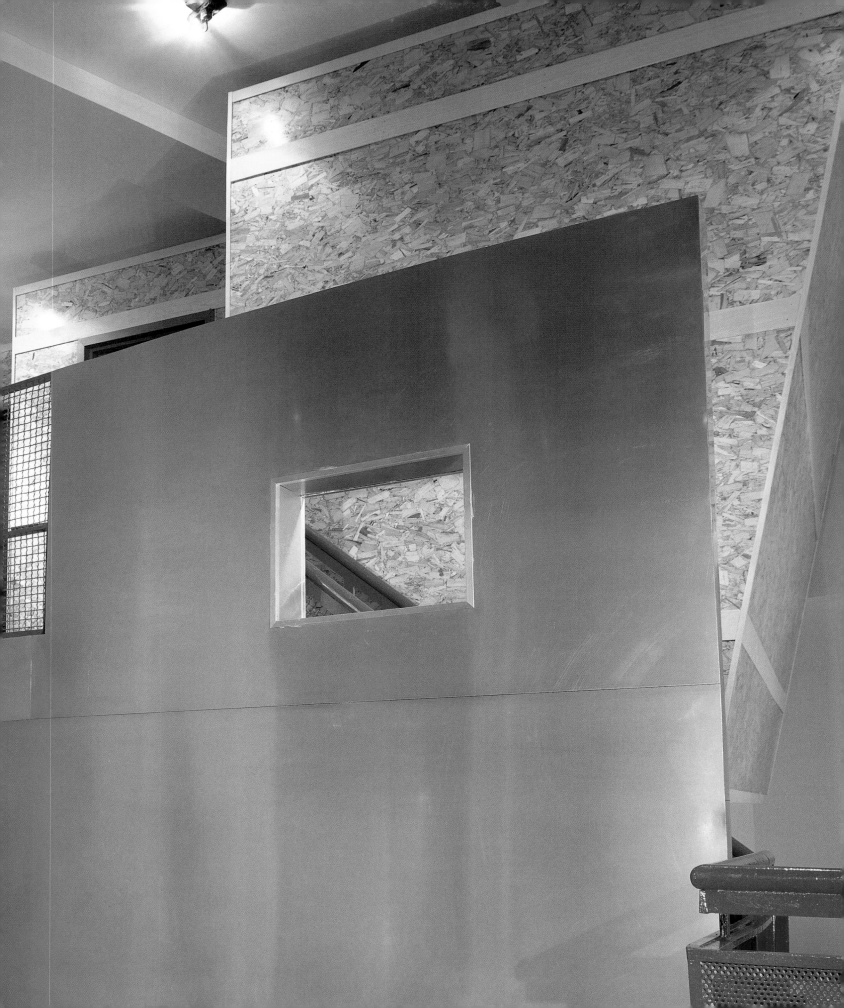

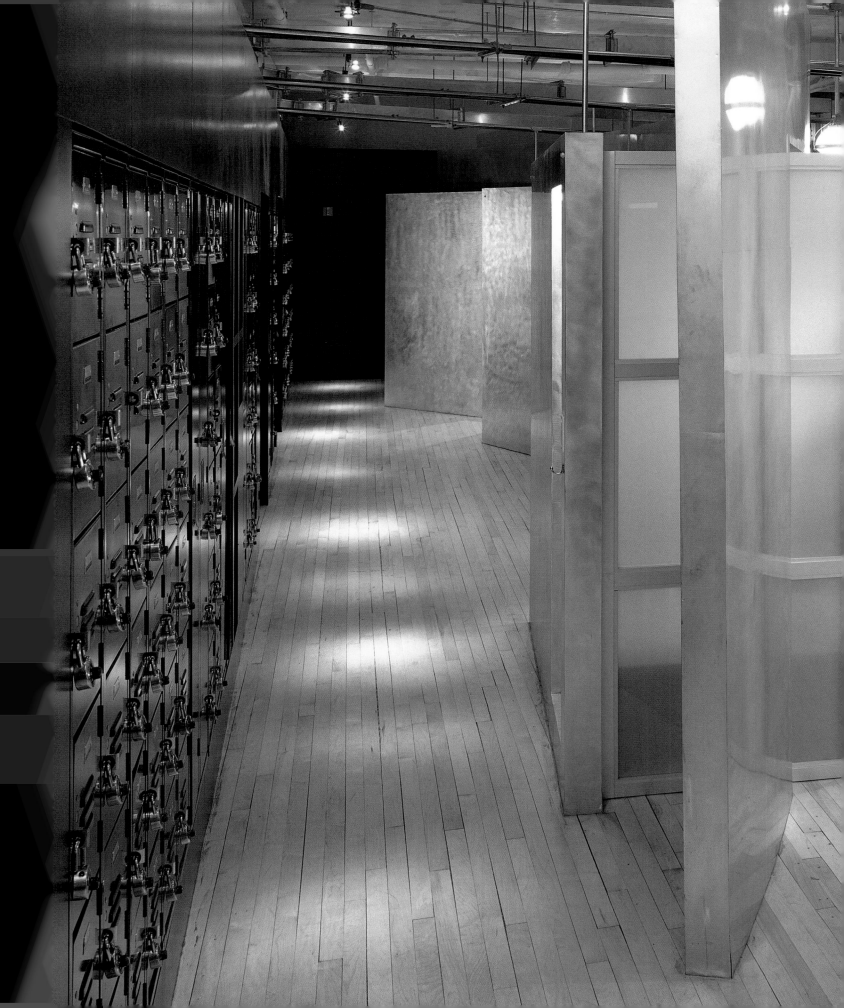

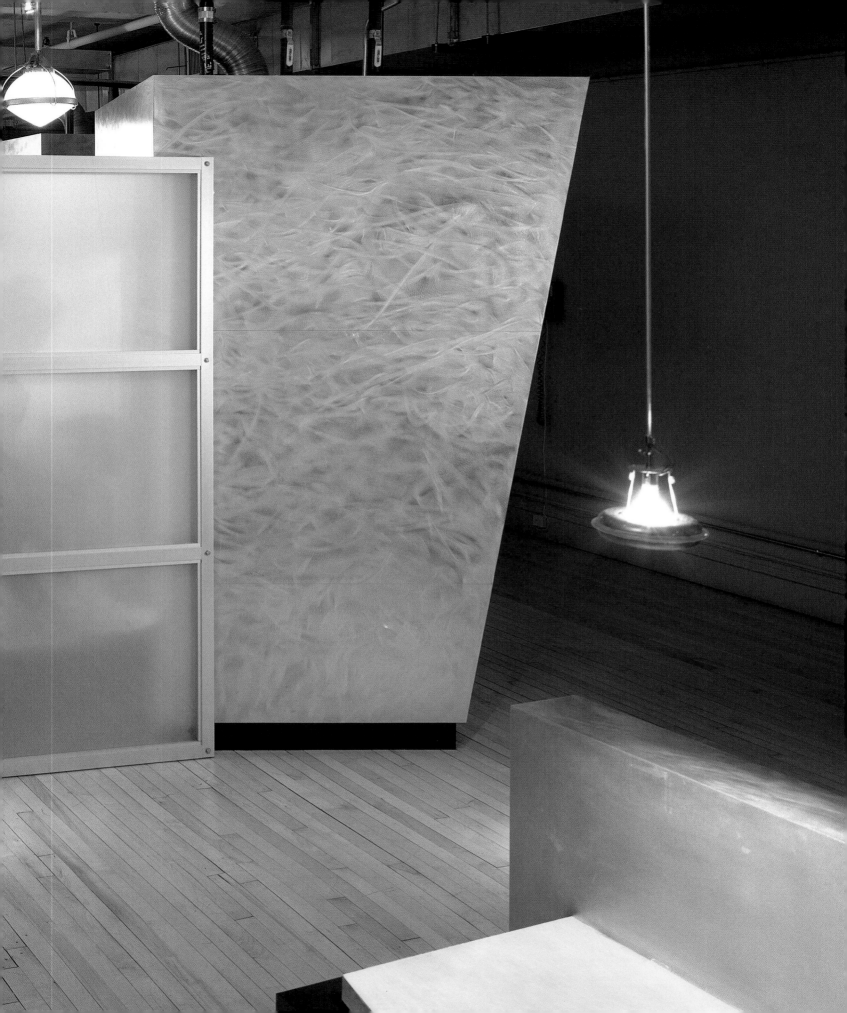

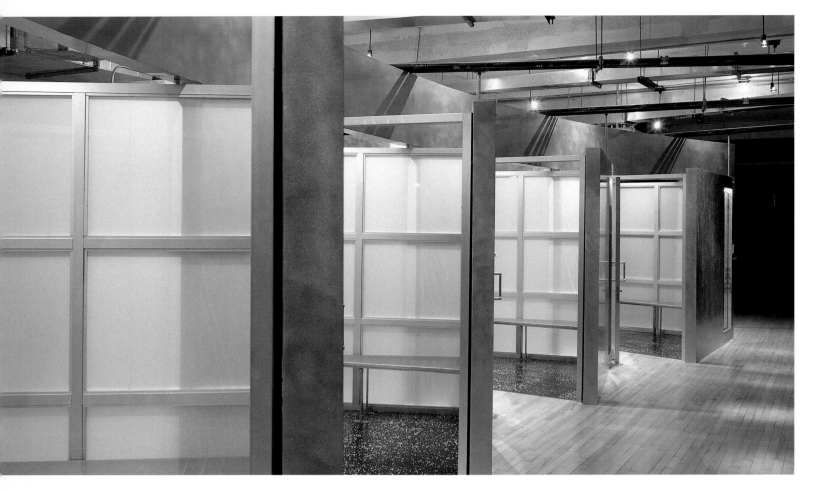

Definitions II

PREVIOUS SPREAD & ABOVE Lines of force are enacted in a curving, copper partition, and angled changing rooms. RIGHT Industrial materials convey strength for little cost. Plumbing lines, ducts, and electrical lines were left exposed as a metaphor for "exposed" bodies. OPPOSITE In contrast to the "exposed" intent of the gym's architecture, the back features a womb-like, enclosed space for massages.

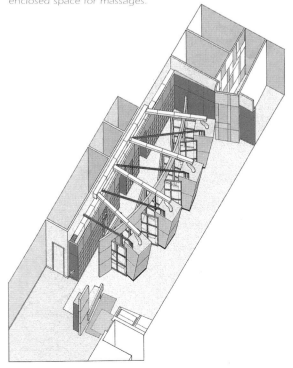

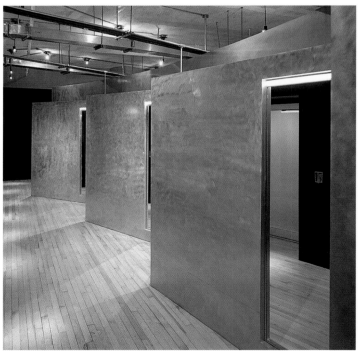

location: **New York, New York**
architect/interior designer: **Thanhauser & Esterson Architects P.C.**
photographer: **© Brian Rose**
square feet/meters: **4,500/418**
design budget: **$400,000**

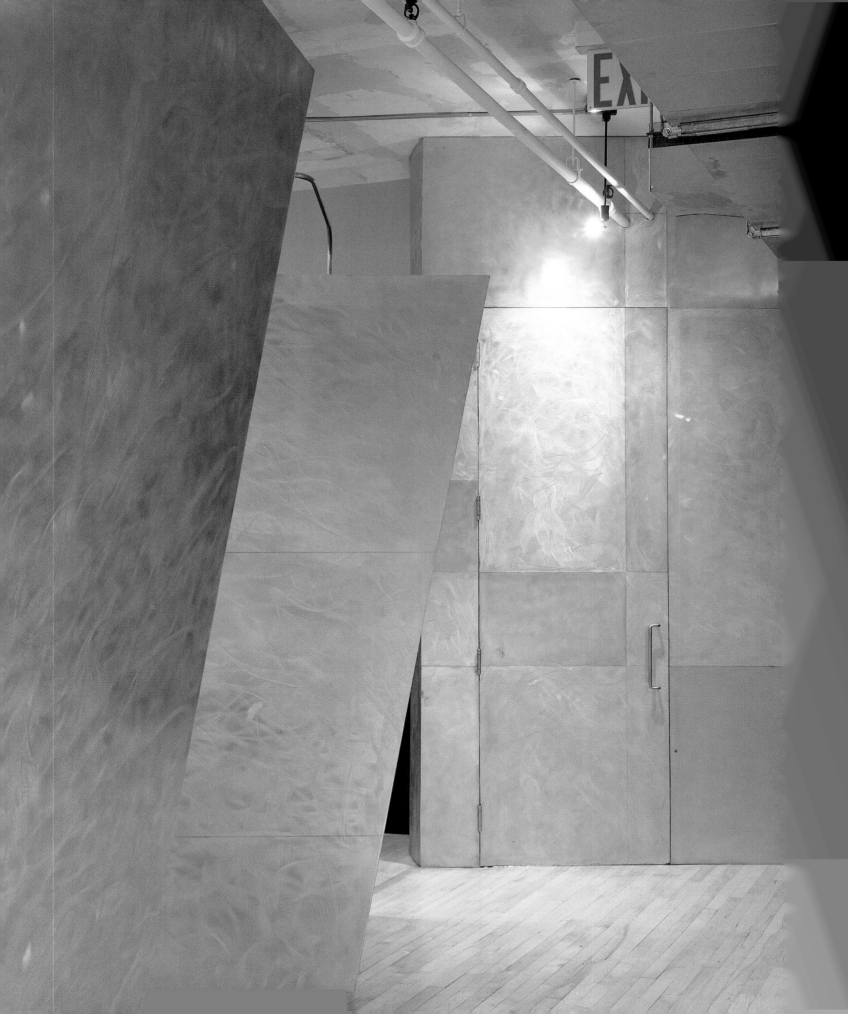

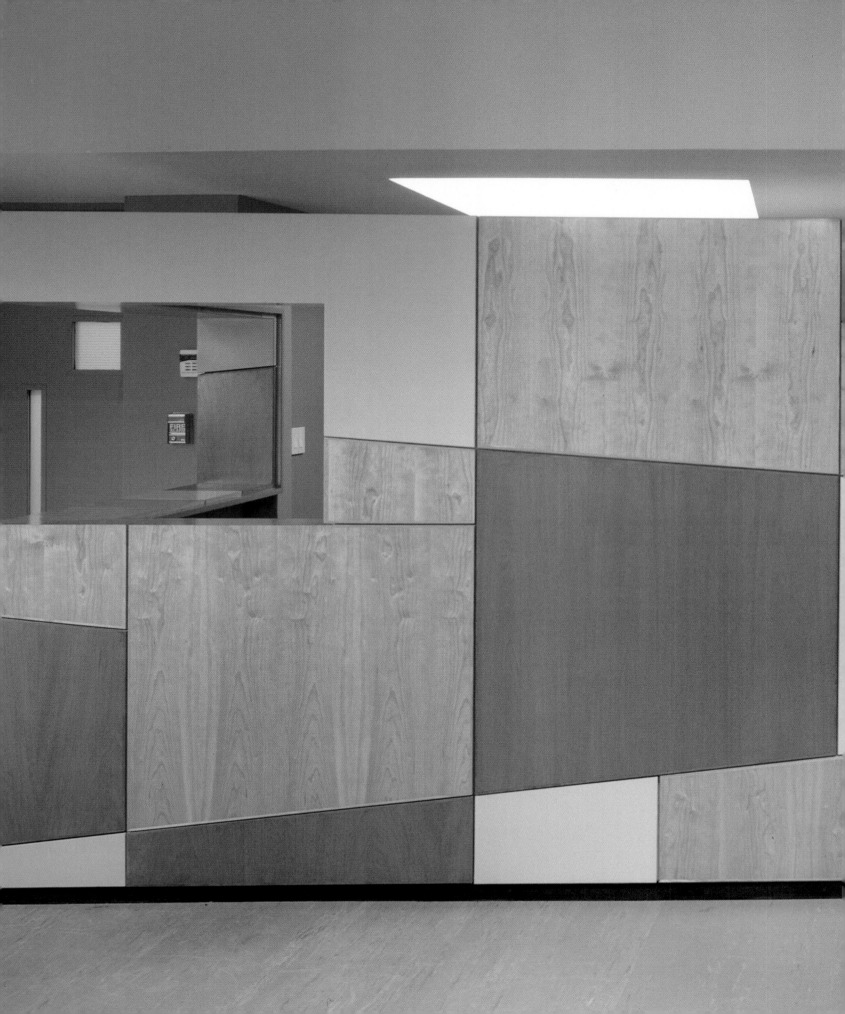

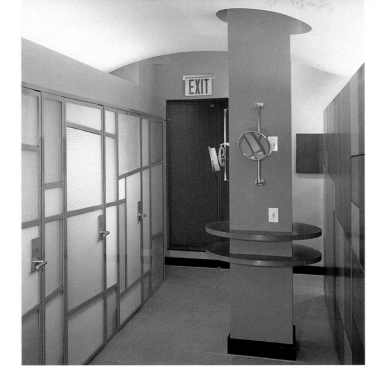

Definitions III

OPPOSITE Sculptural millwork elevations serve as partitions; one houses the reception desk. LEFT The changing room wall, composed of three types of glass, echoes the partition. CENTER LEFT A billowing light sculpture lends a sense of motion to the small, awkward space. BELOW LEFT Steel lockers create bold black horizontals amidst the cool millwork. BELOW In the lacquered steel and glass changing rooms, backlighting creates silhouettes of users that animate the space.

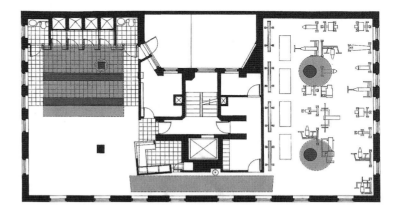

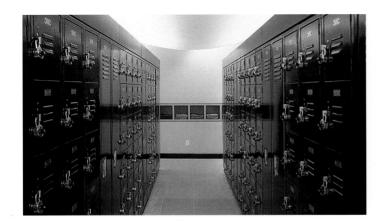

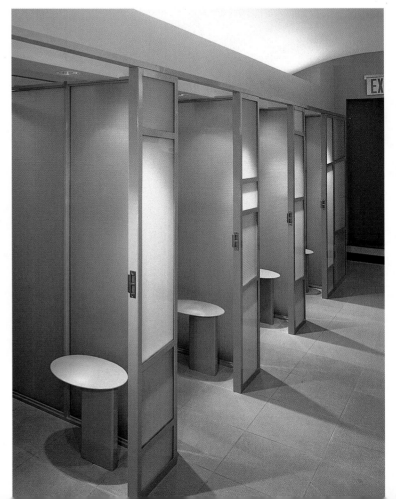

location: **New York, New York**
architect/interior designer: **Thanhauser & Esterson Architects P.C.**
photographer: **© Brian Rose**
square feet/meters: **4,000/372**
design budget: **$500,000**

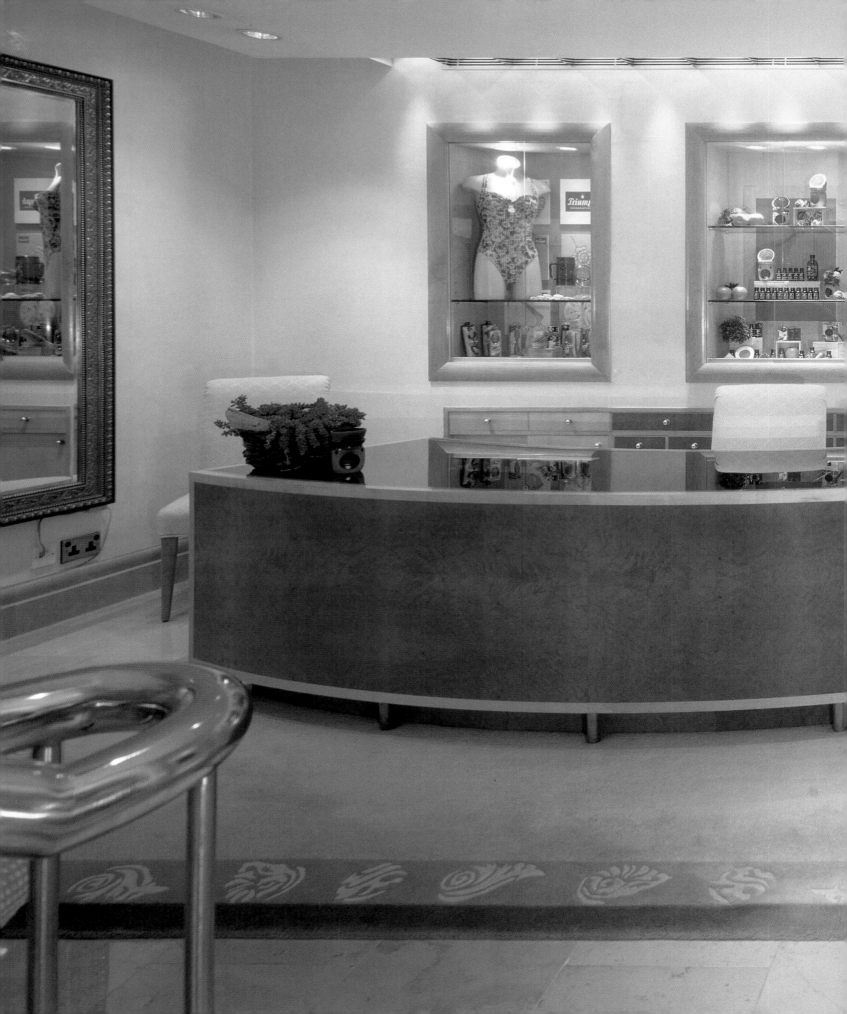

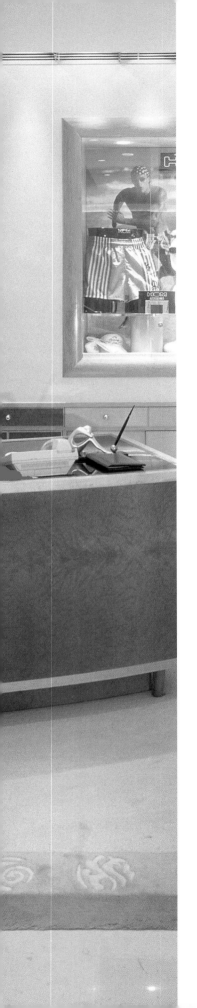

The Peninsula Hong Kong Spa is a decidedly luxurious retreat. Since the hotel found that fitness centers primarily attract Western guests and beauty facilities are preferred by Asian guests, it required a spa that would appeal to both in their five-star style. Design firm Denton Corker Marshall endeavored to accommodate patrons from the super fit to the occasional user, without alienating or intimidating either; the solution was to surround sophisticated equipment with comfortable, intimate interiors.

Active and passive body treatments divide the spa into gymnasium and beauty salon. A grand reception area features a classically themed, patterned-marble floor, sculptured columns, and a rotunda with painted murals and skylights. The level of detail in the changing rooms rivals that of the guest suites, with saunas clad in Norwegian cedar, polished-stone 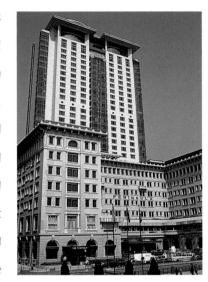 steam baths, and spas tiled in mosaic and gold leaf finish. A grand curved staircase leads to the pool terrace. The sun-filled gymnasium, with its polished wood surfaces and padded fabric walls, provides a range of equipment under vaulted ceilings, and expansive views of the harbor. The Clarins salon off the reception area features massage and facials, among other treatments. Lighting is soft and warm; a subdued color palette with accents of red and blue mosaic offers richness and texture. The Peninsula's business and leisure guests have both been charmed by this urban oasis.

THE PENINSULA HONG KONG SPA

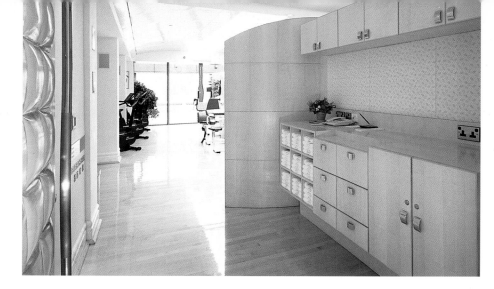

PREVIOUS SPREAD The spa is housed in the penthouse of The Peninsula's new building, offering the classicism of the old hotel with new materials and details. A small retail area is located at the spa's entrance. RIGHT The gymnasium features wood floors, fabric-padded walls, and a wealth of natural light. CENTER & BELOW RIGHT The reception area of the Clarins salon features marble floors, buttery walls, and red accents. Classical "columns" are inspired by the building's architecture. OPPOSITE The whirlpool and plunge pools are tiled in blue mosaic, and are overlooked by a hand painted ceiling with an aquatic scene.

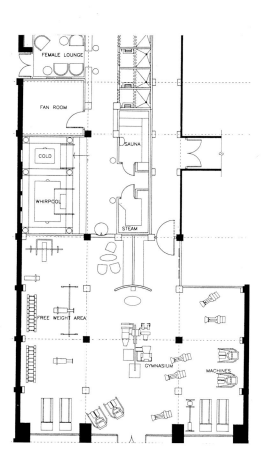

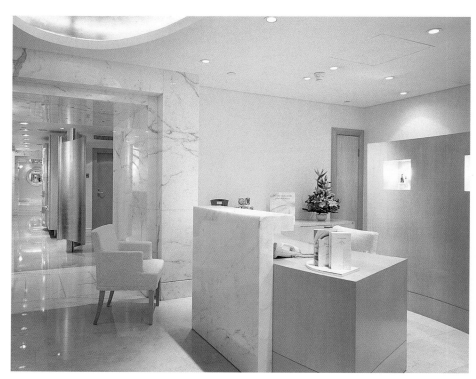

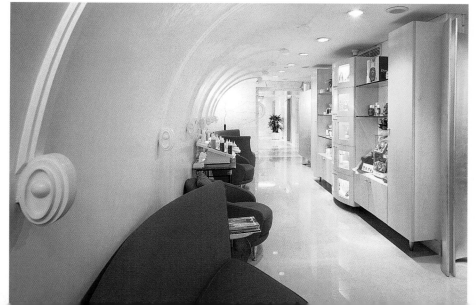

location: Hong Kong, China
architect: Rocco Design Limited
interior designer: Denton Corker Marshall Ltd.
photographer: Hans Schlupp, Australia
square feet/meters: 9,000/836
design budget: not disclosed

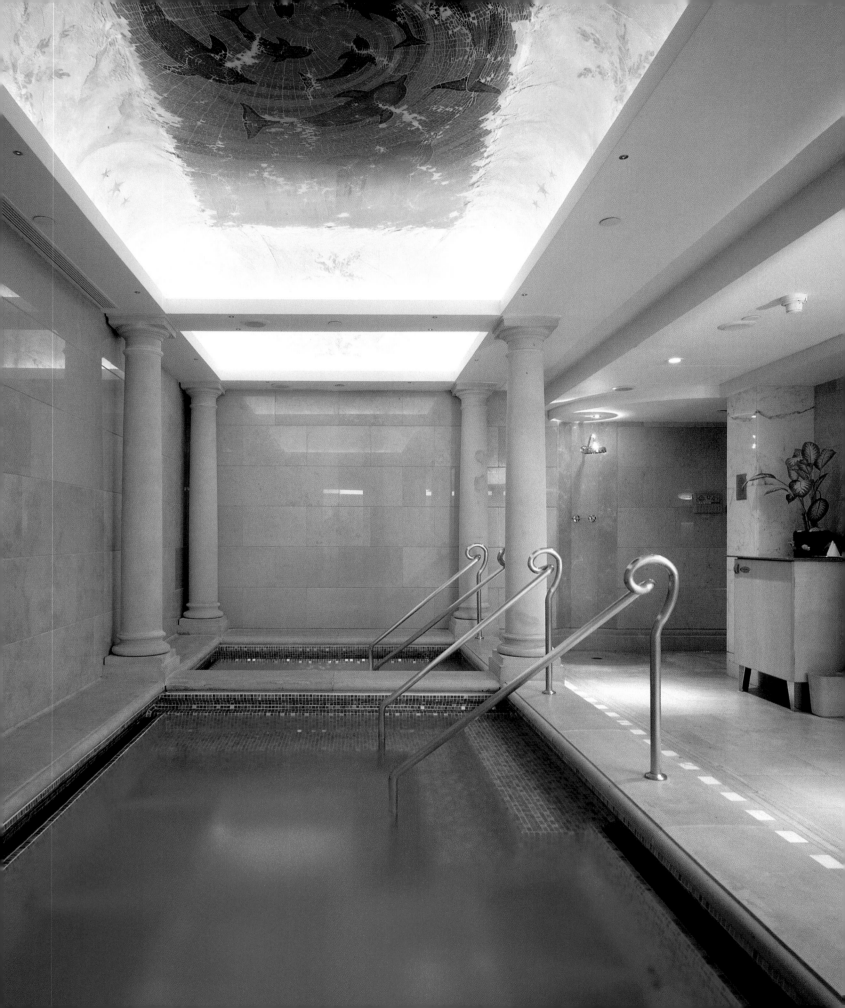

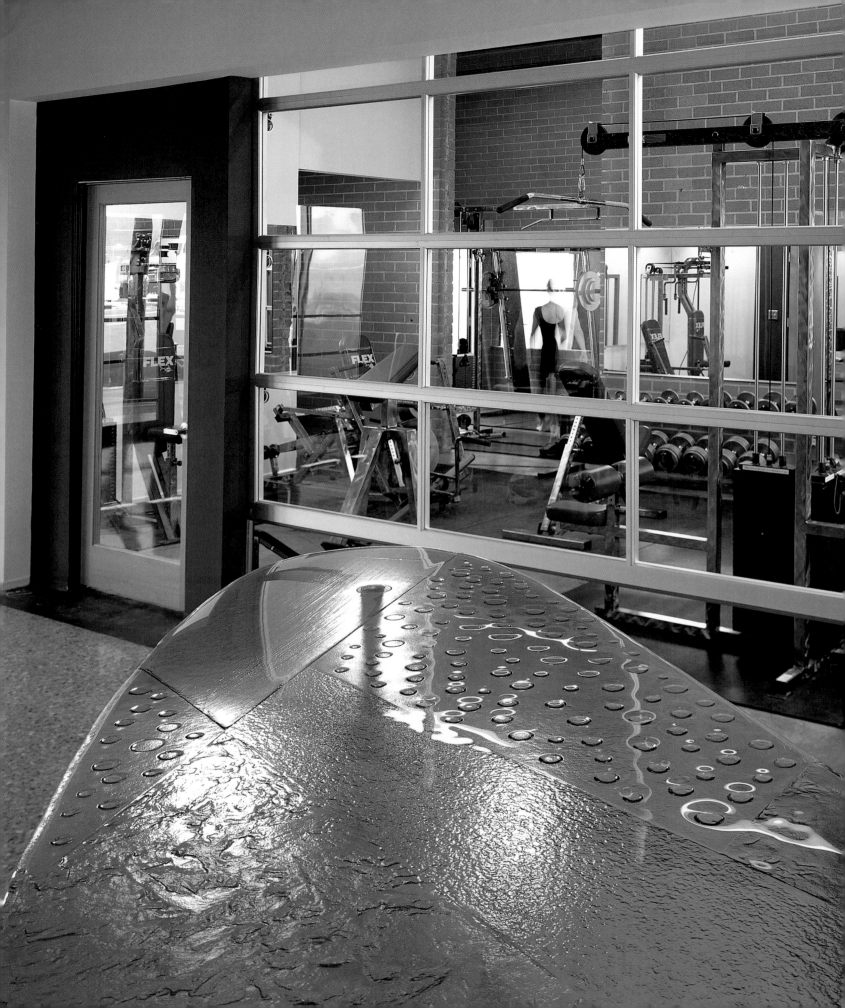

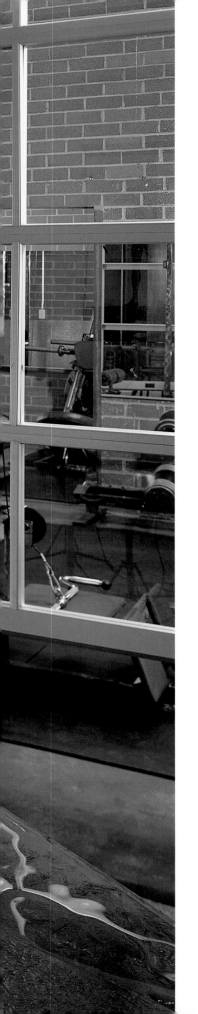

The large illuminated Greyhound sign over the Santa Monica, California bus terminal is a local icon. But when Greyhound decommissioned the terminal a few years ago, salvation came from an unlikely source. Physical trainer Brian Cinadr was persuaded by one of his clients, architect Steven Ehrlich, that it would be perfect for his planned fitness center. By naming the club BUS Wellness Center, Cinadr was able to keep the time-honored sign which is much larger than today's zoning laws would allow.

Working on a shoestring budget, Ehrlich relied on the building's basic elements, removing a drop ceiling to expose the tapered steel roof frame, uncovering the windows and clerestory along the facade, and restoring the brick walls and terrazzo floor. A new main corridor from sidewalk to rear parking lot provides order and natural light, and doubles as a rest-aurant. All amenities open off

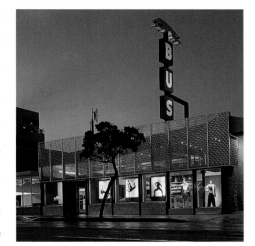

this central passage: check-in, retail area, kitchen, aerobics studio, free weights and stretching areas, Pilates method areas, and locker rooms. The studio and gyms can be enclosed with roll-down glass doors, or left open; skylights provide natural ventilation. A new wood and steel fin was inserted to stabilize the aerobics room, but most of the structure already conformed to state seismic code. A cast-glass serving counter and black-and-white photographs were commissioned from local artists.

BUS WELLNESS CENTER

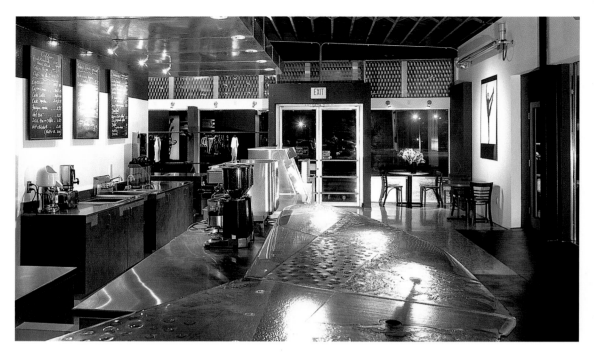

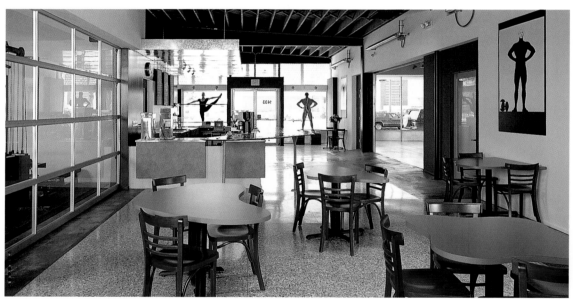

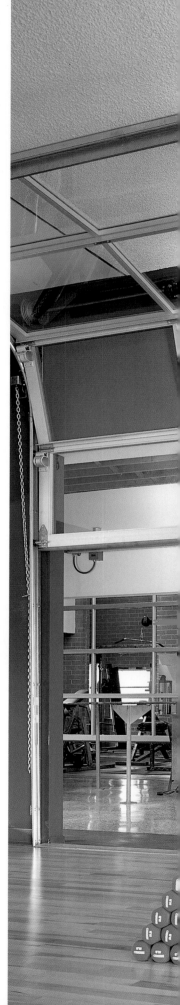

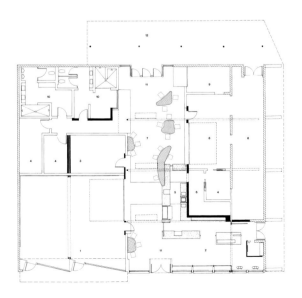

PREVIOUS SPREAD A cast-glass serving counter is one of several commissioned artworks. TOP The architects restored the building's original structure, including the tapered steel roof frame and terrazzo floors. ABOVE For the café, laminated tables were made from cardboard templates. RIGHT A roll-down glass door either exposes or partitions the aerobics studio.

location: Santa Monica, California
architect/interior designer: Steven Ehrlich Architects
photographer: Adrian Vilecescu, AV Media
square feet/meters: 5,360/498
design budget: $200,000

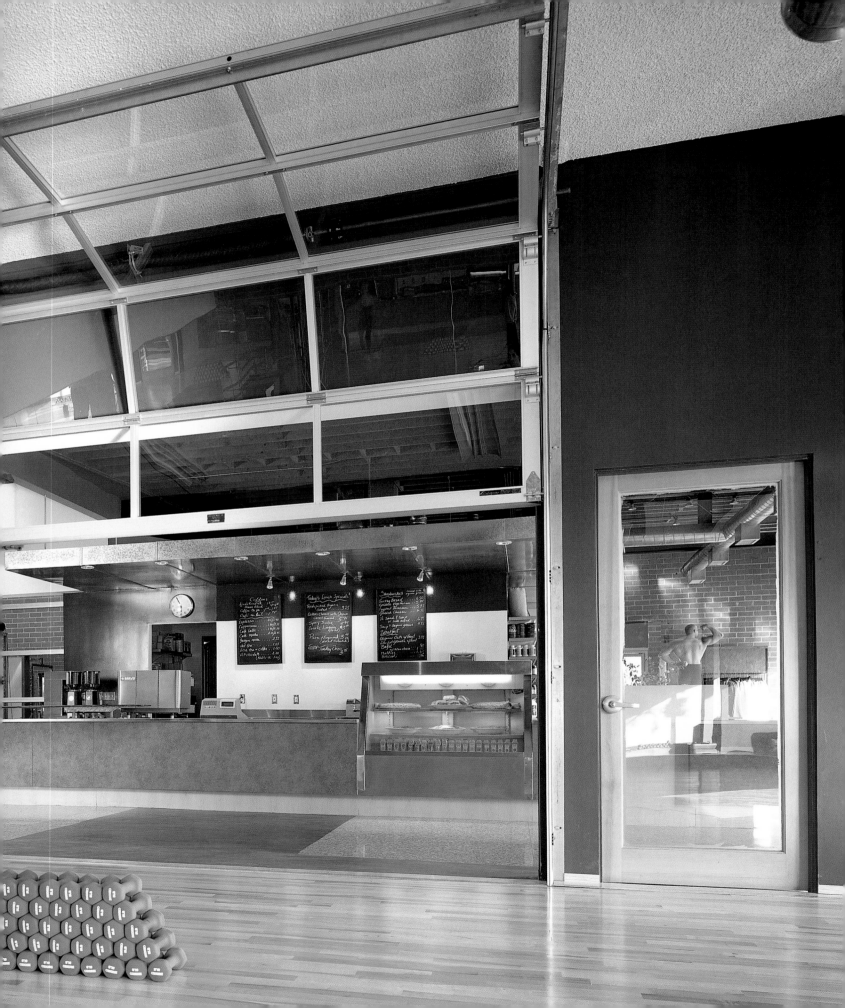

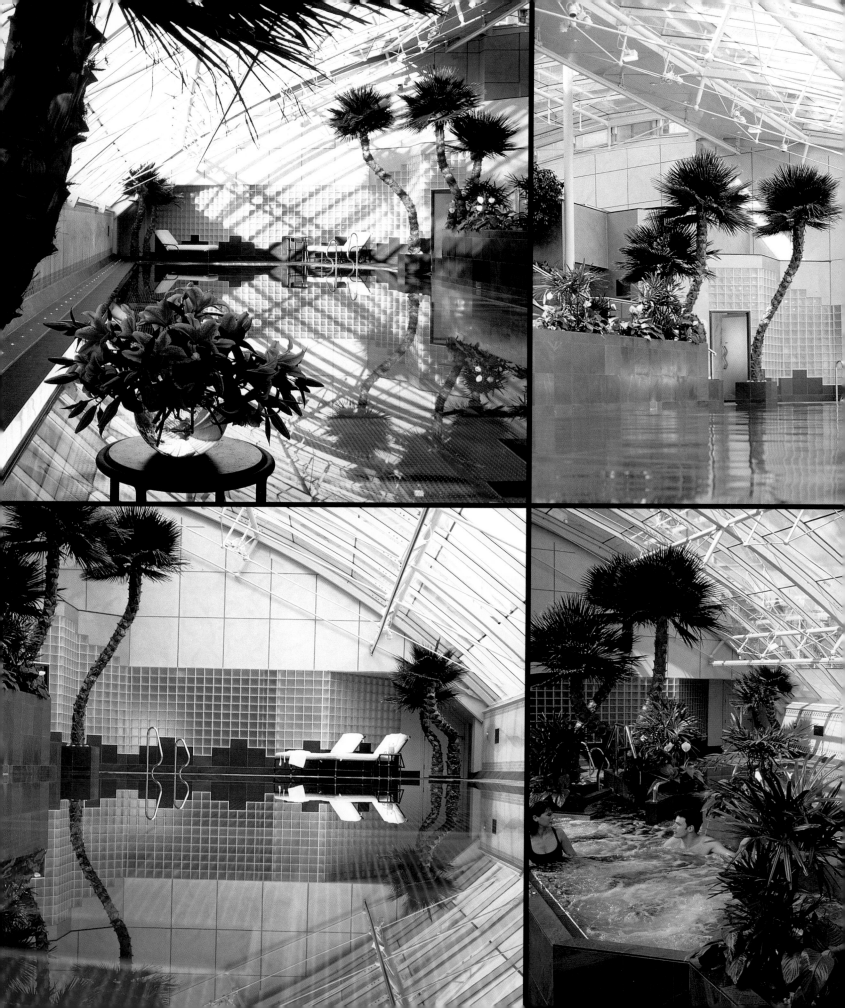

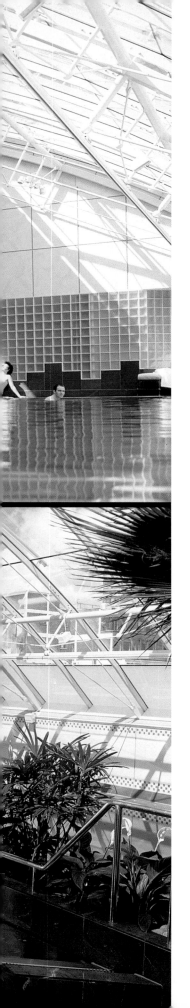

H irsch/Bedner Associates' classic contemporary design for the Peak, a Hyatt Health Club, appeals to both guests of the Hyatt Carlton Tower and residents of its upscale Cadogan Place neighborhood in London. The challenge was to create a comfortable atmosphere that matched the hotel's sleek interiors and fit gracefully in a tight space.

The health club is located on two floors linked by a panoramic elevator: the exercise and massage rooms are on the ninth floor (top level), with pool and spa treatment rooms on the second; both locations feature locker rooms. The natural focal point of the ninth floor incorporates breathtaking views of the city. The bright, sun-filled space offers cardiovascular and strength training equipment, and an aerobics studio alongside the more sybaritic Club Room bar and restaurant. On the second floor, the luxurious glass-roofed pool, water garden, and conservatory

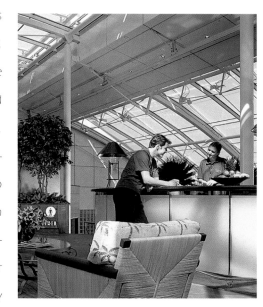

update the health club and offer a hip, social space. A stunning 20-meter stainless steel pool and whirlpool are lined with palms and greenery; amenities include a sauna, steam room, sun bed, and Clarins beauty salon. Simple materials such as glass block, stainless steel, slate, rattan, and wood create a soothing, timeless retreat.

THE PEAK A HYATT HEALTH CLUB

PREVIOUS SPREAD The stainless steel pool is lit by a glass roof and lined with palm trees. Greenery and natural materials such as rattan and frosted glass lend a greenhouse atmosphere. A whirlpool overlooks the pool from a tree-lined perch. RIGHT An expansive glass roof, walls, and partitions create a sense of openness. BELOW Comfortable pool chairs and a private seating area allow for relaxing and socializing. BELOW RIGHT The women's locker room features sinks and mirrors centered around a palm tree as an exotic touch. OPPOSITE From the lounge, where members can browse through newspapers, to the healthy cuisine of the restaurant, the Club Room area provides an elegant respite.

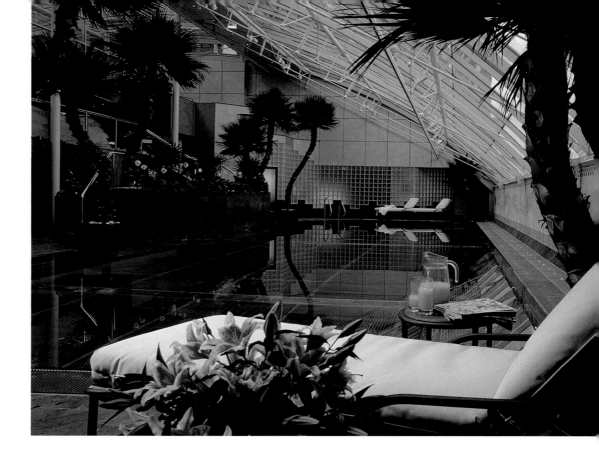

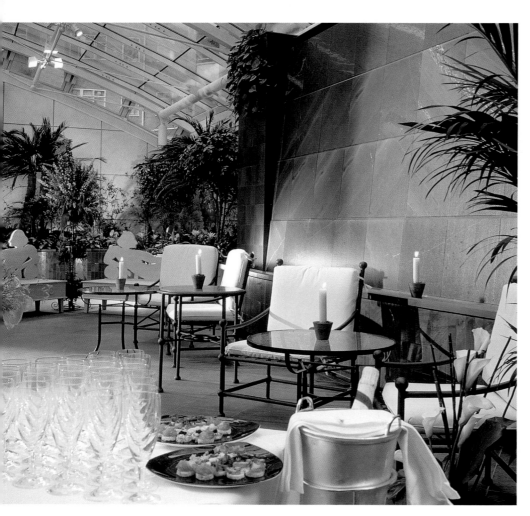

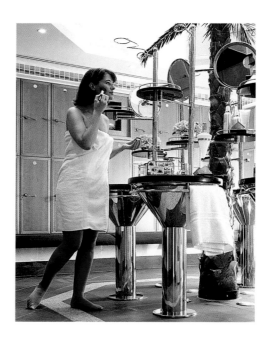

location: **London, England**
architect: **Colwyn Foulkes & Partners**
interior designer: **Hirsch/Bedner Associates**
photographer: **Ken Kirkwood, London**
square feet/meters: **13,994/1,300**
design budget: **$3 million**
club membership: **1,200**

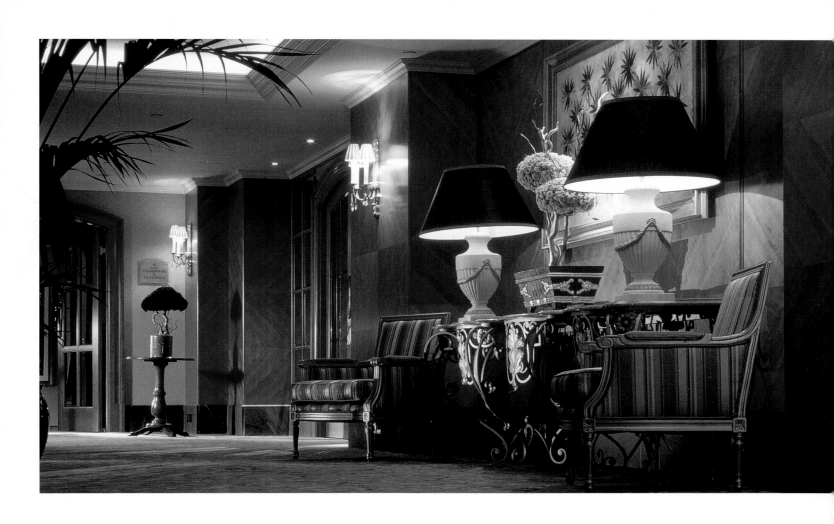

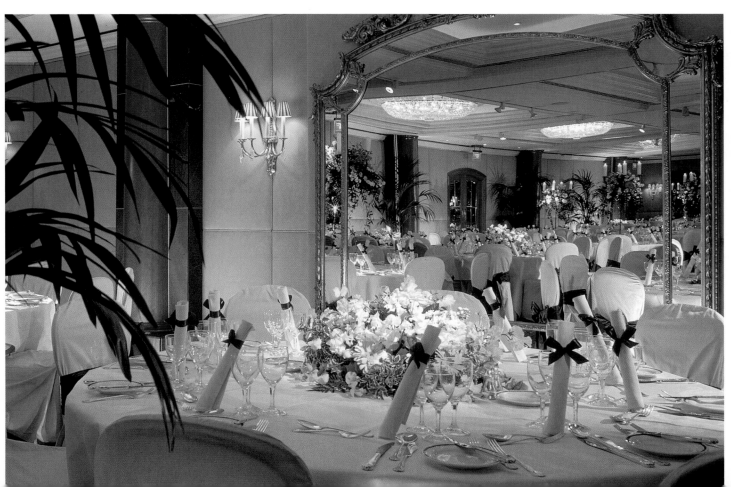

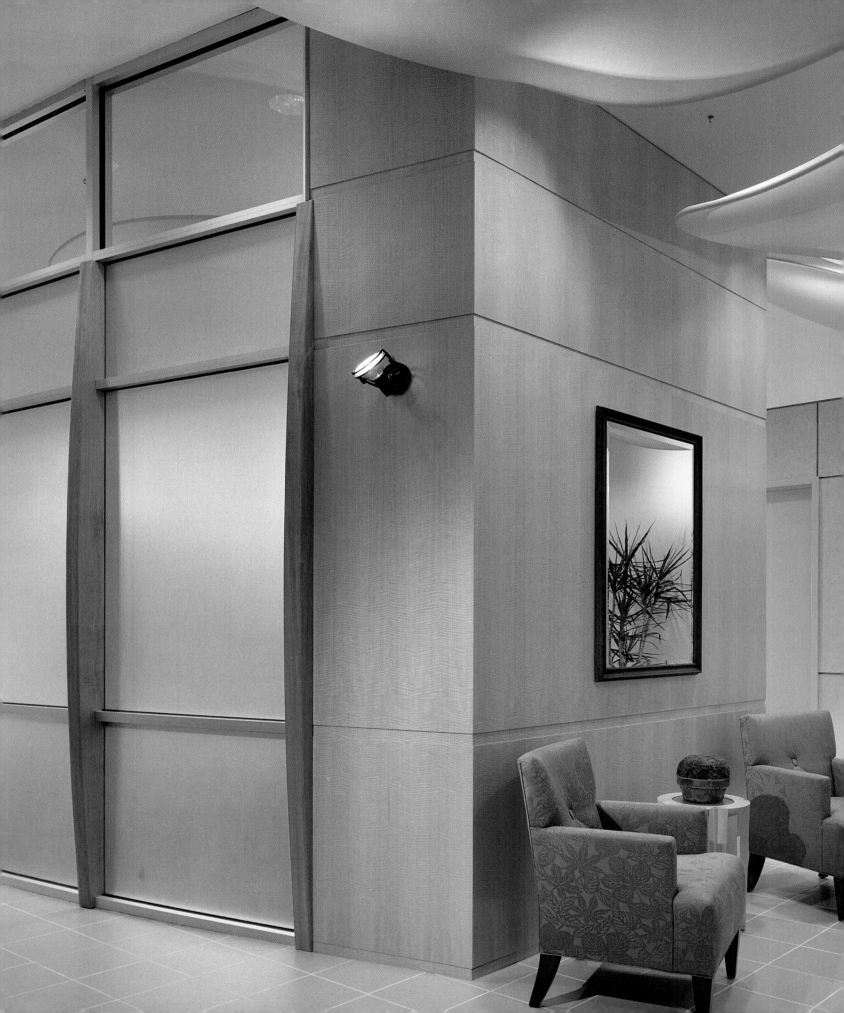

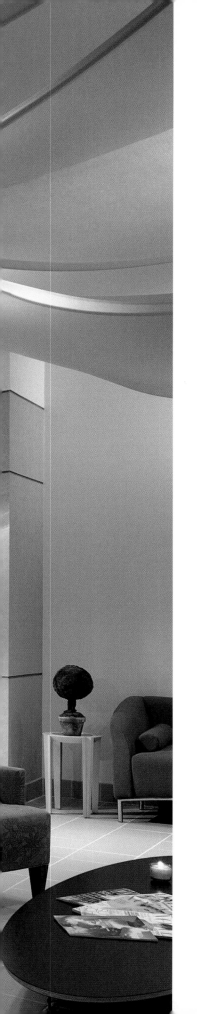

M any of today's top hotels are transforming their spa facilities from an afterthought to a focal point. For example, renovations of the Spa at Short Hills were intended to increase guest room and restaurant revenues, and attract a large local membership. Design director William W. Whistler of Brennan Beer Gorman Monk/Interiors likens the spa's new interiors at the Hilton at Short Hills to "the healthy glow achieved at the end of an aerobic workout or body treatment, with a clean color palette and minimalist decor with as few lines as possible."

Featured are a new entrance/reception area, ten massage and wet therapy rooms, two facial rooms, a cardiovascular/weight-training room and aerobics studio, and a juice bar. The pool area and locker rooms were also expanded. In the weight-training room, natural light streams in through 13-foot-high windows, supported by ambient

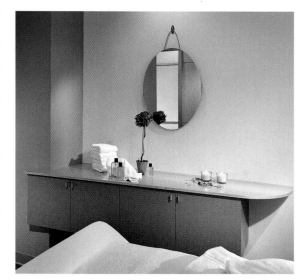

lighting and a sunbaked color palette. Wood framed mirrors mimic the window mullions for classical symmetry, while the massage and facial area is elliptical in plan with sleek, curved wood and glass walls. Massage rooms offer contemporary furnishings, and stretched fabric canopies conceal ceiling light fixtures for an even, subdued effect.

THE SPA AT SHORT HILLS

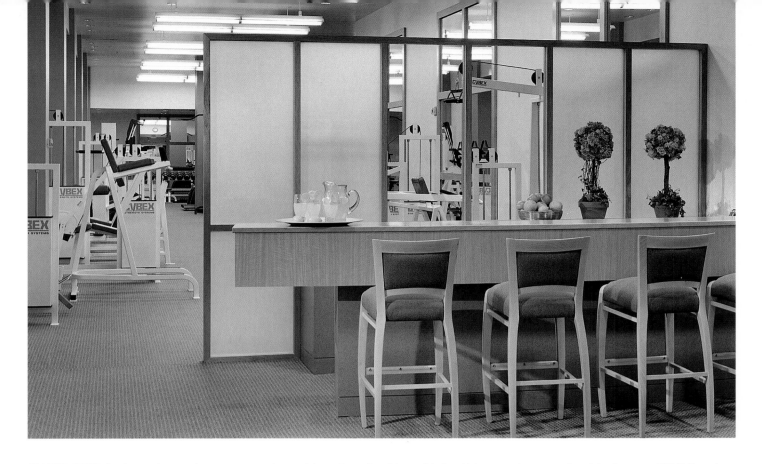

PREVIOUS SPREAD In the spa's reception area, natural materials and comfortable, stylish furnishings create a warmly minimal space. ABOVE The glass-paneled juice bar offers a respite from the cardiovascular/training area. BELOW In the cardiovascular area, floor-to-ceiling windows are echoed by mullioned mirrors for classical symmetry. OPPOSITE The massage rooms are sleek yet calming spaces, offering simple elements and subtle lighting.

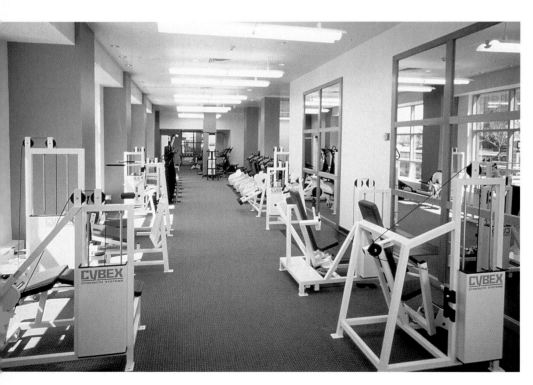

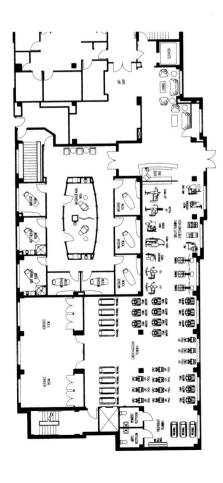

location: **Short Hills, New Jersey**
interior designer: **Brennan Beer Gorman Monk/Interiors**
photographer: **Paul Warchol**
square feet/meters: **16,000/1,486**
design budget: **$1 million**

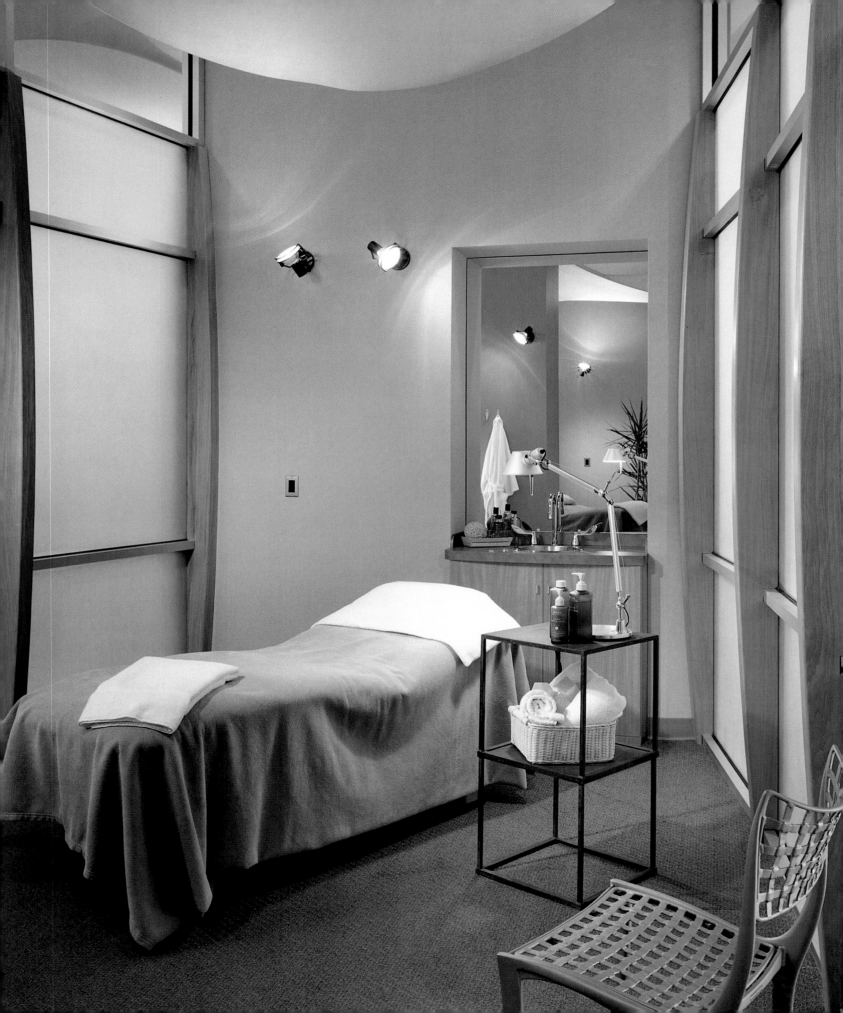

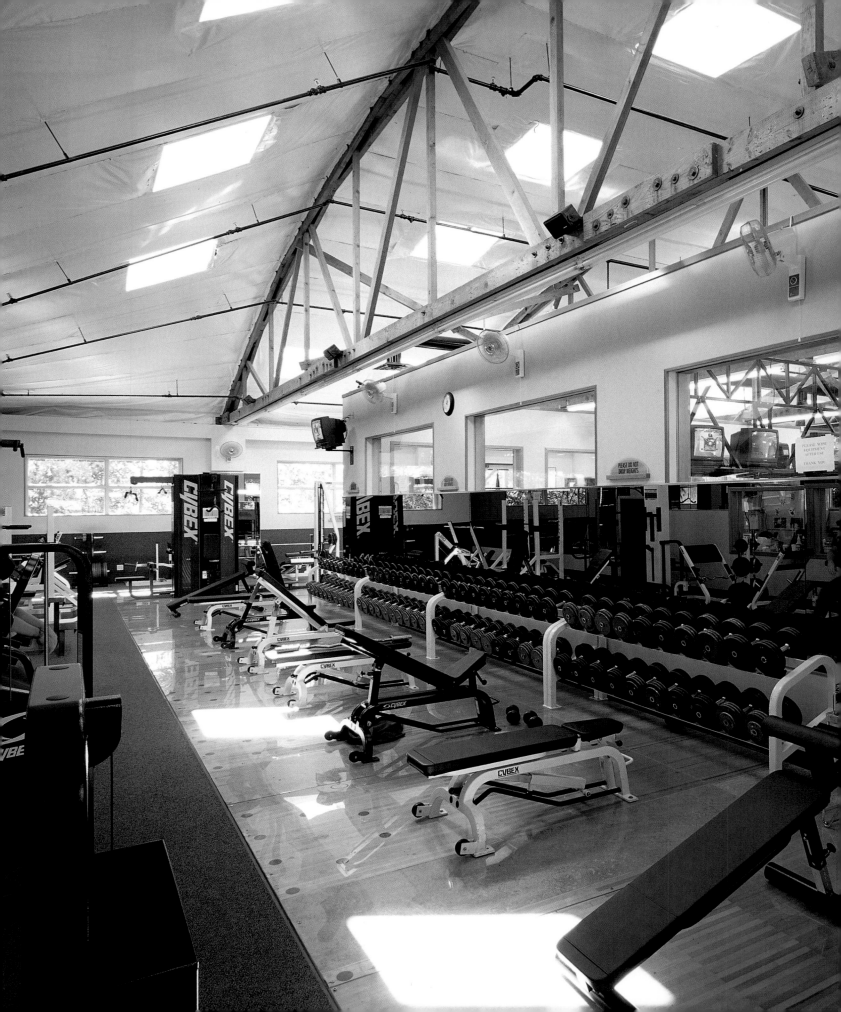

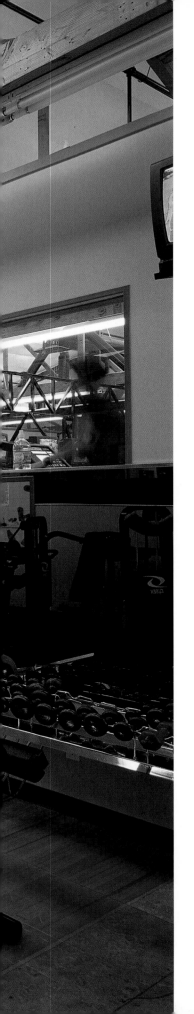

P art medical clinic, art gallery, and Internet salon, Bainbridge Health Maintenance Center proudly suffers a bit of an identity crisis. Located on Bainbridge Island, Washington, in a community of about 18,000, the club quickly outgrew its original basement facility. A former '40s bowling alley—that era's health club—proved to be the perfect contemporary milieu, as redesigned by O'Connor Associates. Working with interior designer Gale Martin, the dropped ceilings and bowling fixtures were removed to expose original timber trusses and maple floors. Windows and skylights were introduced, creating an alluring blend of exposed structure, organic materials, and natural light.

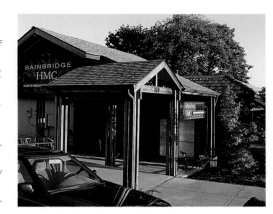

The layout of the 14,000-square-foot club is tightly defined. To provide transition, the main workout space is at a lower level than the entry and locker rooms. At its core is a partitioned cluster of medical and physical therapy offices, and a large cardiovascular room; the workout circuit wraps around the perimeter and leads to the weightlifting and stretching areas. The designers' goal to provide a variety of visual stimuli includes artwork, mirrors, windows, and individual televisions, as well as Internet and e-mail access.

Bainbridge Health Maintenance Center's roster of amenities is impressive: it is a national test site for Cybex equipment, offers babysitting, numerous seminars, and integrates internal, sports, and naturopathic medicines, as well as chiropractic and physical therapies. A juice bar and spa are planned.

BAINBRIDGE HEALTH MAINTENANCE CENTER

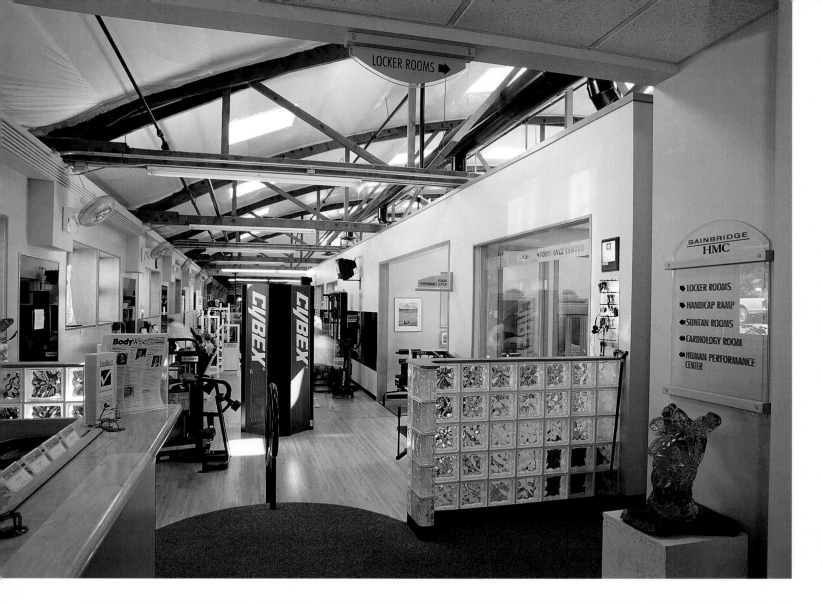

PREVIOUS SPREAD Bainbridge Health Maintenance Center features the original timber trusses and maple floors. Natural light is introduced through windows and skylights. ABOVE The workout space is set at a lower level than the entry to provide a sense of transition. Medical offices are located in a partitioned central core. Natural light penetrates the club through skylights, glass walls, and floating partitions that define smaller spaces underneath the massive roof. BELOW The cardiovascular equipment is also at the core of the space, with free weights and stretching areas wrapped around it. OPPOSITE Artwork is integrated throughout the club to offer additional visual stimuli.

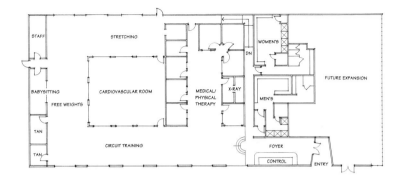

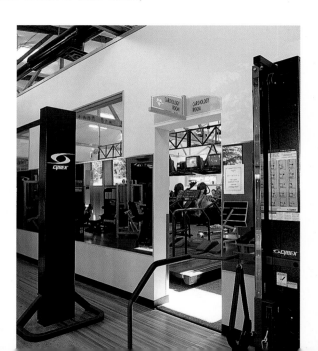

location: Bainbridge Island, Washington
architect: O'Connor Associates
interior designer: Gale Martin
photographer: Art Grice
square feet/meters: 14,000/1,301
design budget: $1.62 million
club membership: 5,000

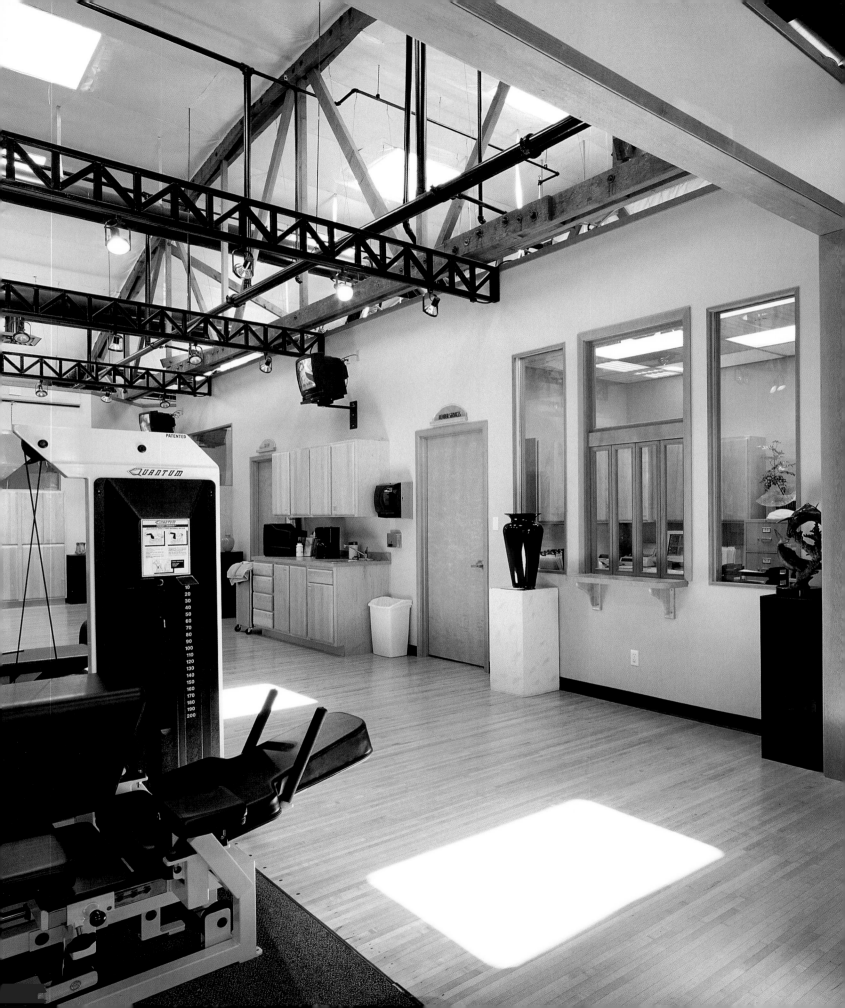

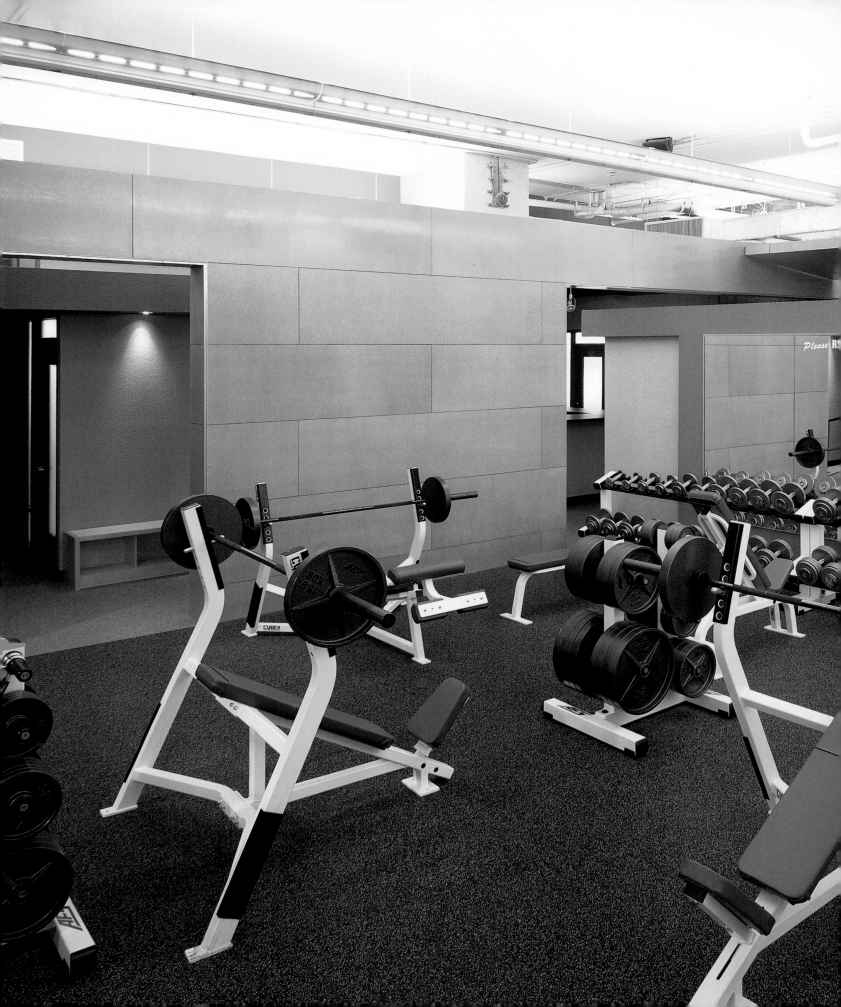

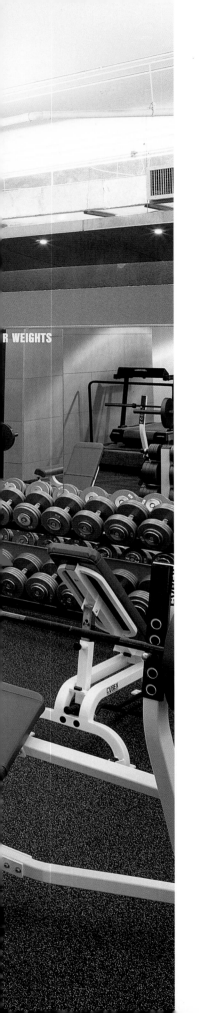

L ocated in a two-story space at the base of a Florida office building, *Premier Health & Fitness* is an energetic, visually alive space, created by Resolution: 4 Architecture. The designers defined the gym's diverse programmatic needs—cardiovascular and weight training, massage, aerobics, and nutrition—and combined the disparate activities into a unified conception of fitness.

Brightly colored, monolithic walls modulated by openings make visual and circulatory connections between zones. The dance of colors, openings, and planes frames different visual compositions, depending on one's vantage point. Kiosks housing the membership offices, a retail area, and juice bar are carved into the space, further encouraging movement throughout.

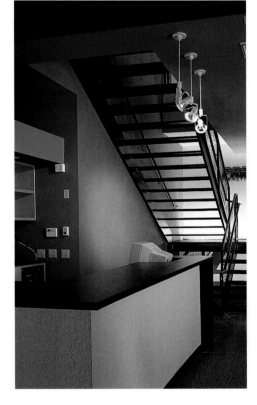

The surfaces reflect the designers' interest in bringing off-the-shelf materials into a refined environment. Walls consist of lacquered fiberboard and textured gypsum board; a raked, low plywood ceiling defines a main corridor. Lighting is softened by inverting hung industrial fixtures to face the ceiling. An illuminated landing and surrounding soffits and openings add drama to the steel staircase.

PREMIER HEALTH & FITNESS

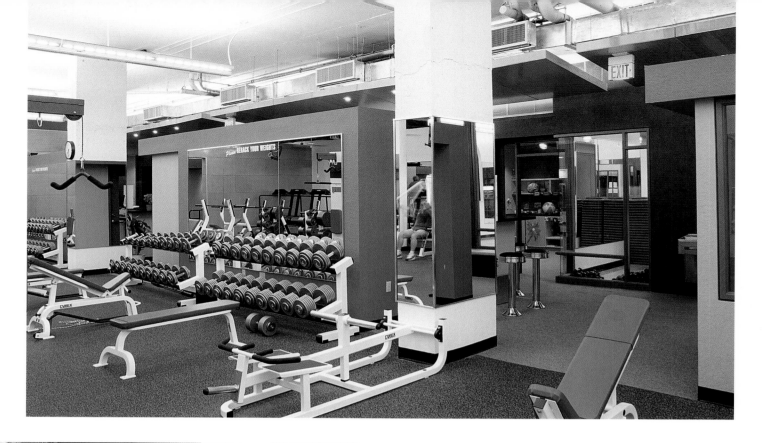

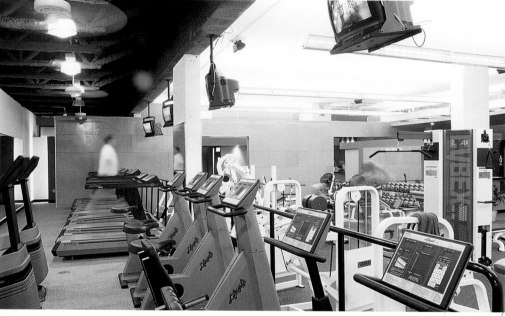

PREVIOUS SPREAD The interior is a lively composition of planes, colors, and passages. **ABOVE** Public and private areas are defined by zones. **LEFT** Sunny walls and carefully adjusted light fixtures evenly illuminate the fitness stations. **OPPOSITE** The designers employed abundant color to energize and diversify the workout space.

location: **Hallandale, Florida**
architect/interior designer: **Resolution: 4 Architecture**
photographer: **© Thomas Delbeck**
square feet/meters: **16,000/1,486**
design budget: **$500,000**
club membership: **1,000**

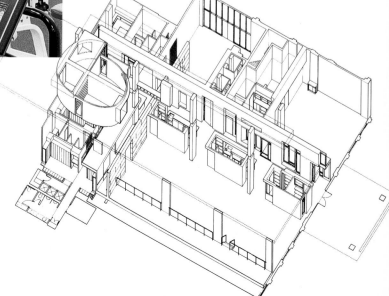

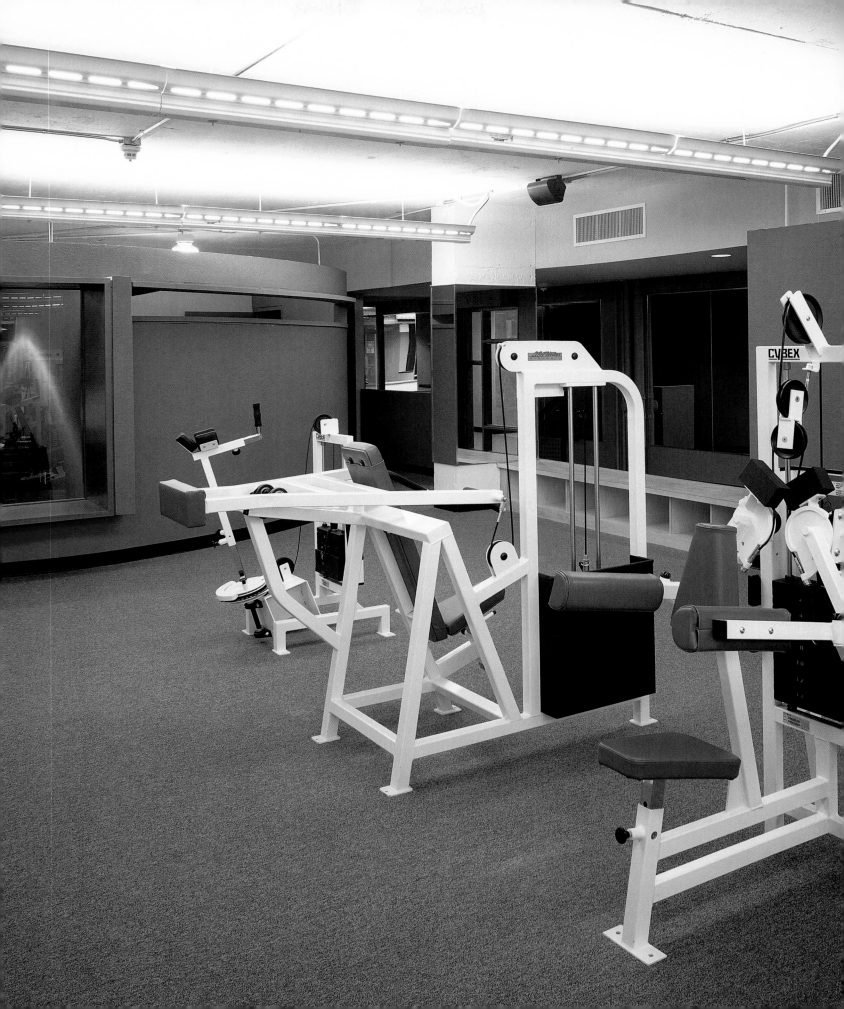

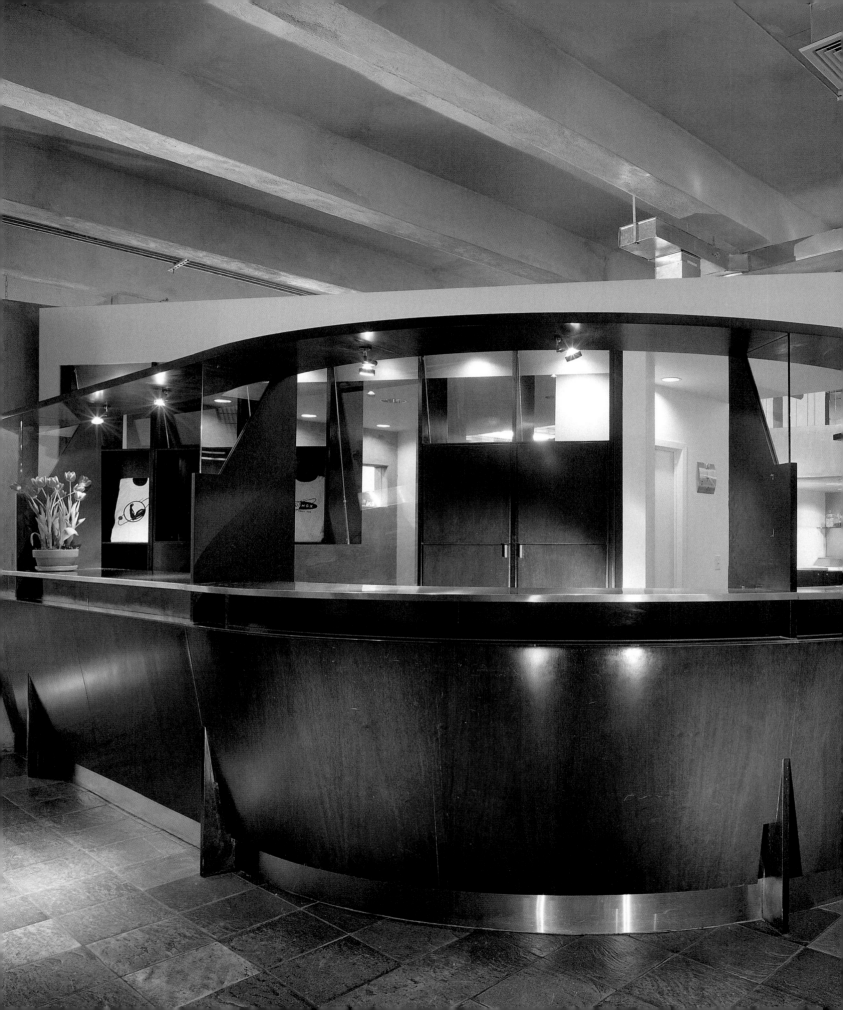

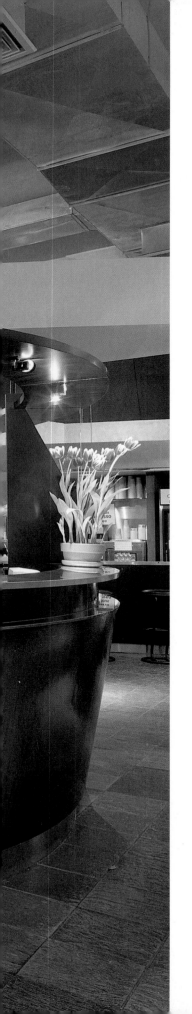

M ojo Stumer Associates' designs for the first two Equinox Fitness Clubs could be considered the first to successfully target and attract Manhattan's throngs of young professionals. "The concept was to change the image of a health club with a cutting edge, contemporary design," says Mark Stumer, offering clients the high-end environment they were used to demanding of their restaurants, retail stores, and apartments.

For the first club, formerly a supermarket on the Upper West Side, the low ceilings were removed and the concrete structure left exposed for a feeling of space. This industrial theme extends to the fixtures and finishes: brushed aluminum panels and stair rails, copper-panel partitions, and steel mesh soffits and reception desks. The urban-inspired palette of grays and blacks is accented by cherry panels, while mats, carpeting, and locker rooms display shades of blue and purple. Behind the retail

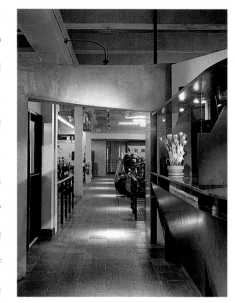

and food areas, which are open to the public, the carefully ordered layout offers cardiovascular equipment on all three levels. Free weights and machines occupy levels one and three, aerobics and spinning rooms are on level two, and locker rooms are stationed on both the first and second floors. An adjacent spa is complete with massage and therapy facilities. The uptown club won an American Institute of Architects Award, and led to Mojo Stumer Associates' design of the next installation.

EQUINOX FITNESS CLUBS

The second Equinox Fitness Club perfectly suits its downtown Manhattan location, where photography, fashion, and design professionals commingle. Housed in a landmark structure offering four levels of workout facilities, the lofty space combines clean lines, industrial materials, and period details. The main double-height workout space, defined by the restored columns, features weight training and stretching areas on the first floor, overseen by a mezzanine of cardio-vascular facilities. A lower level offers additional weight training, testing and nutrition rooms, as well as physical therapy and massage clinics. An airy, loft-like top level features natural light streaming through oversized windows. The color palette is a subtle black, white, and gray, accented by panels in hot tones to signal the reception areas and locker rooms. Industrial-style fixtures keep it simple: steel mesh panels and floor grates, a massive steel staircase, and glass overhangs. Wood reception and café fixtures are elegantly unadorned. Like its predecessor, the downtown location won an American Institute of Architects Award.

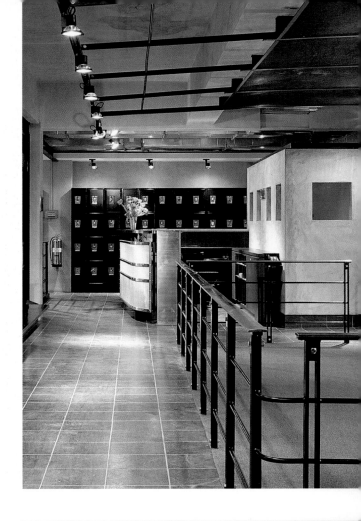

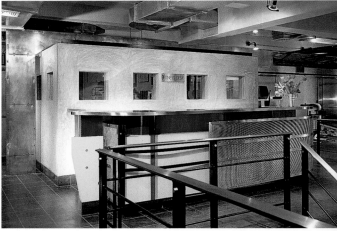

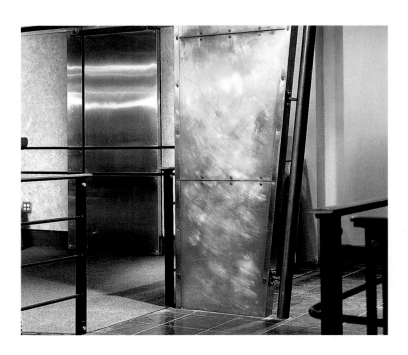

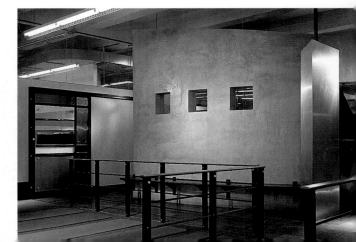

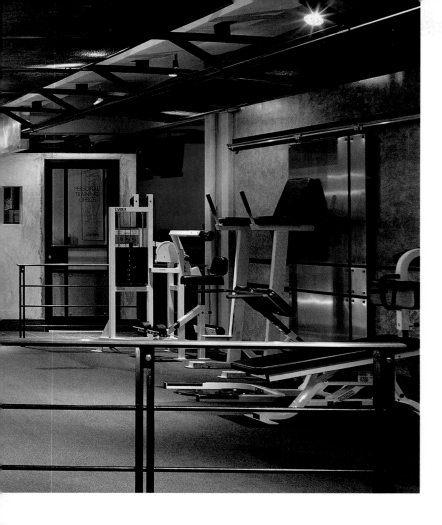

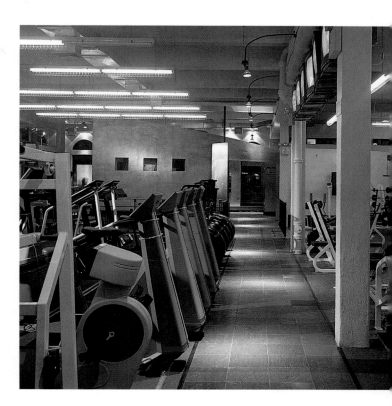

location: **New York, New York**
architect/interior designer: **Mojo Stumer Associates**
photographer: **Frank Zimmerman**
square feet/meters: **12,000/1,115**
design budget: **$600,000**
club membership: **3,000**

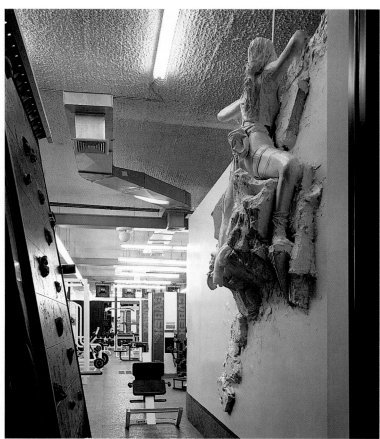

76th Street

PREVIOUS SPREAD The monumental reception desk is a sensuous curving shape, with high-gloss wood veneer as a contrast to the floors and ceilings. The first floor walkway travels through a cardiovascular area, apropos for a club populated by a young New York crowd that likes to see and be seen. **OPPOSITE LEFT** The designers make the most of a column, juxtaposing asymmetry with smooth copper. **OPPOSITE CENTER** At the second floor check-in area, the whole materials palette is visible: untreated stainless steel, brushed aluminum, copper paneling, steel mesh, and injections of hot colors. **OPPOSITE BELOW** A brushed aluminum volume divides the public and reception areas from the front of the workout space. **ABOVE LEFT** The industrial, hard-edge interiors are animated by jewel tones of magenta and blue that signal the second-floor offices and aerobics studio. Lighting is quite low over the stretching area. **ABOVE** Partitions are staggered throughout the space, creating a series of frames. **LEFT** A practice climbing wall is faced by another wall with a life-size sculpture of a climber.

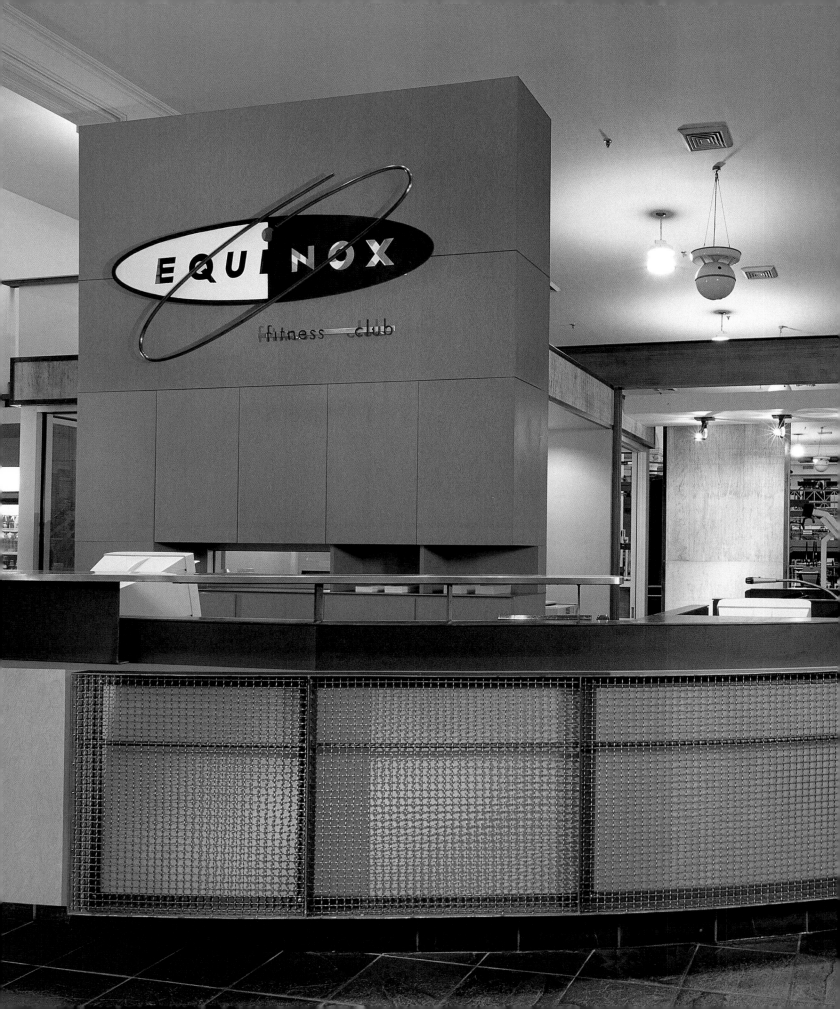

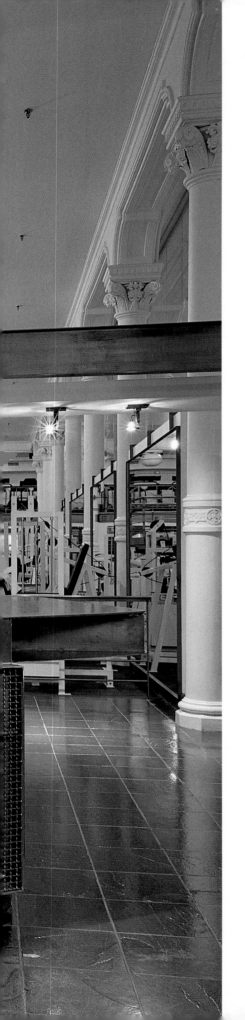

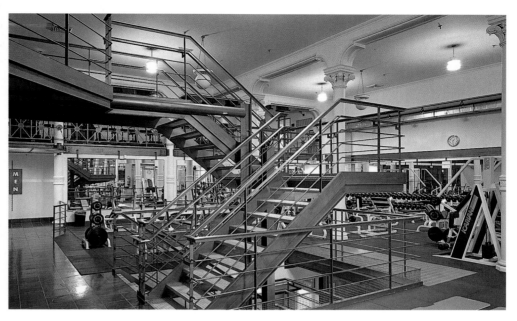

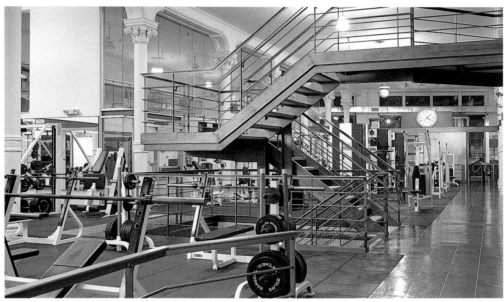

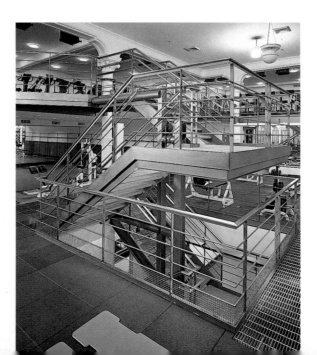

19th Street

FAR LEFT In contrast to the natural palette, tomato-red cabinetry signals the reception area. TOP The soaring double-height main floor creates a loft-like feel that appeals to the Flatiron district neighborhood. ABOVE & LEFT On the main floor is the central weight training area, which acts as a visual stimulus for members using cardiovascular equipment on the mezzanine.

19th Street

RIGHT Original columns in the landmark building were retained to enliven and order the space. CENTER & BELOW RIGHT The sub-grade level features another reception area, for personal training and massage check-in. OPPOSITE LEFT & BELOW The retail area is sited next to the reception desk, and is open (like the café) to members and nonmembers. OPPOSITE ABOVE RIGHT Housed in the steel, glass and mesh "box" is a membership office; to the back are the retail area and an aerobics studio.

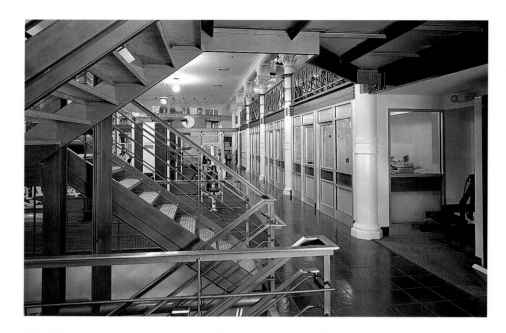

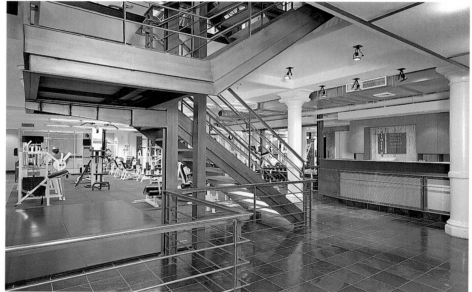

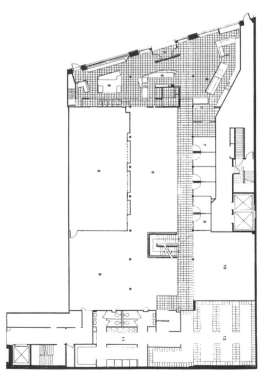

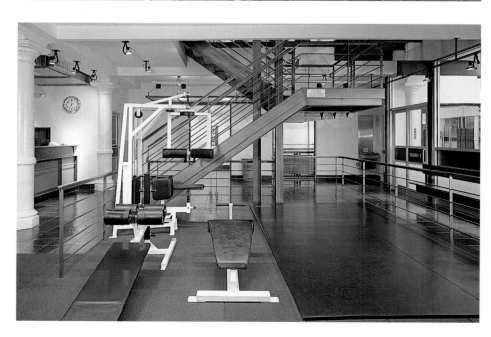

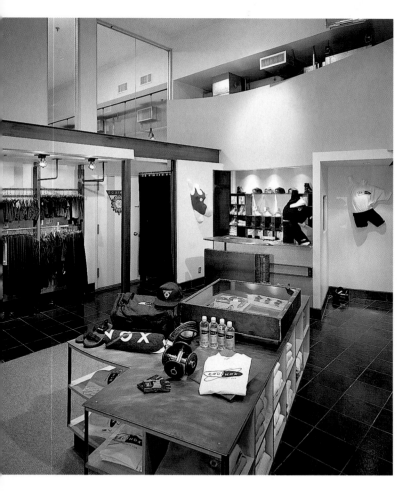

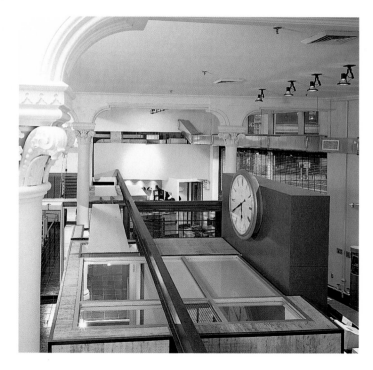

location: **New York, New York**
architect/interior designer: **Mojo Stumer Associates**
photographer: **Frank Zimmerman**
square feet/meters: **20,000/1,858**
design budget: **$1.2 million**
club membership: **10,000**

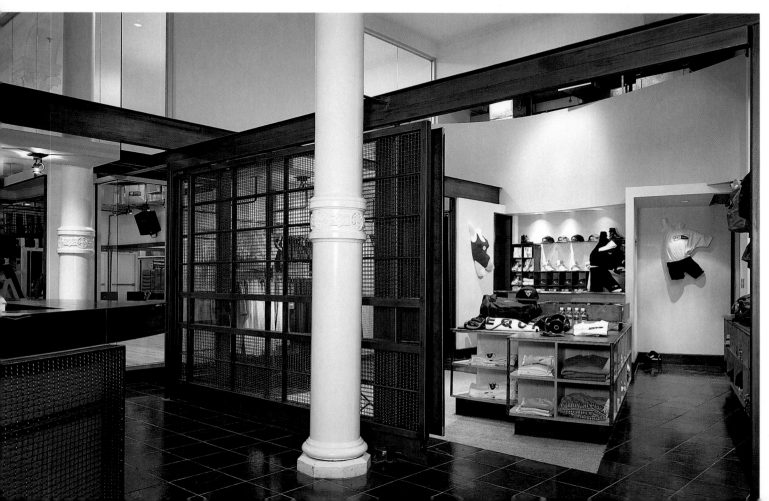

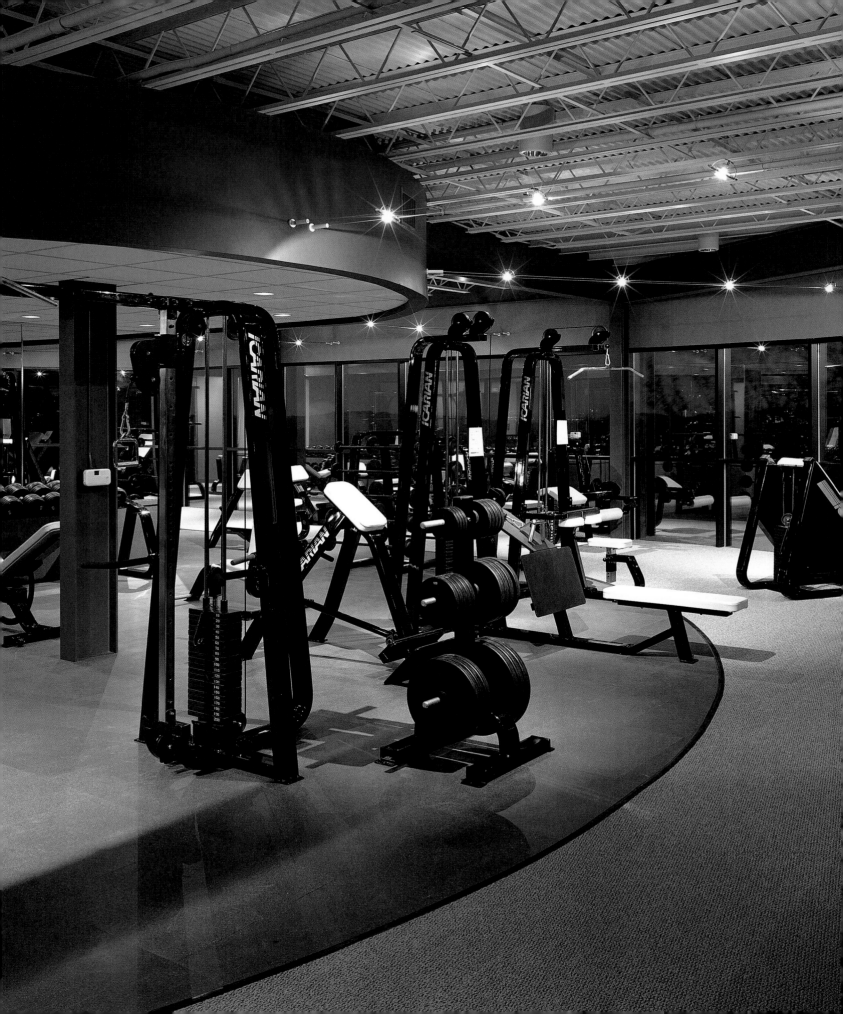

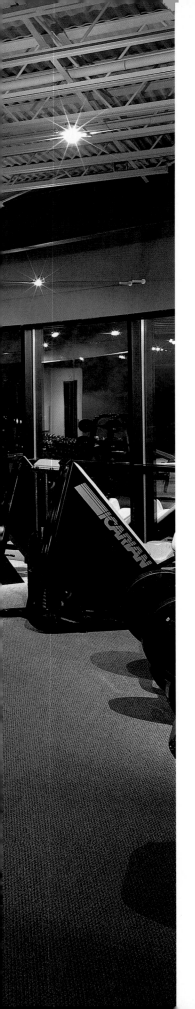

For the interiors of Wild Basin Fitness, Peel Paulson Design Studio took its cue from the club's spectacular hill country surroundings. Natural materials bring the outdoors in, while the abundant views, highlighted with mirrors and lighting, bring the exercisers out.

Peel Paulson simply and stylishly transformed the former commercial space by removing the drop ceilings and installing string lighting and custom light fixtures; unsightly plumbing and electrical panels were disguised by new walls. To create the one-on-one personal training center, the designers left as much workout space as possible, yet allowed for spacious locker rooms, massage areas, and a juice bar. Cardiovascular and strength training areas are separated for quiet and easy traffic flow. Finishes and furnishings are simple in detail, elegant in materials and eye-catching in

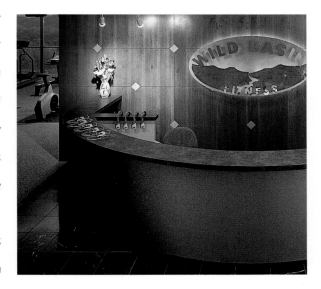

concept. Marble, slate, and limestone surfaces, floor tile patterns, wood lockers and millwork are attractive but unfussy components. Rubber flooring and coated weights, easily cleaned surfaces, and ample space left between machines ensure the safe, serene atmosphere intended by the designers.

WILD BASIN FITNESS

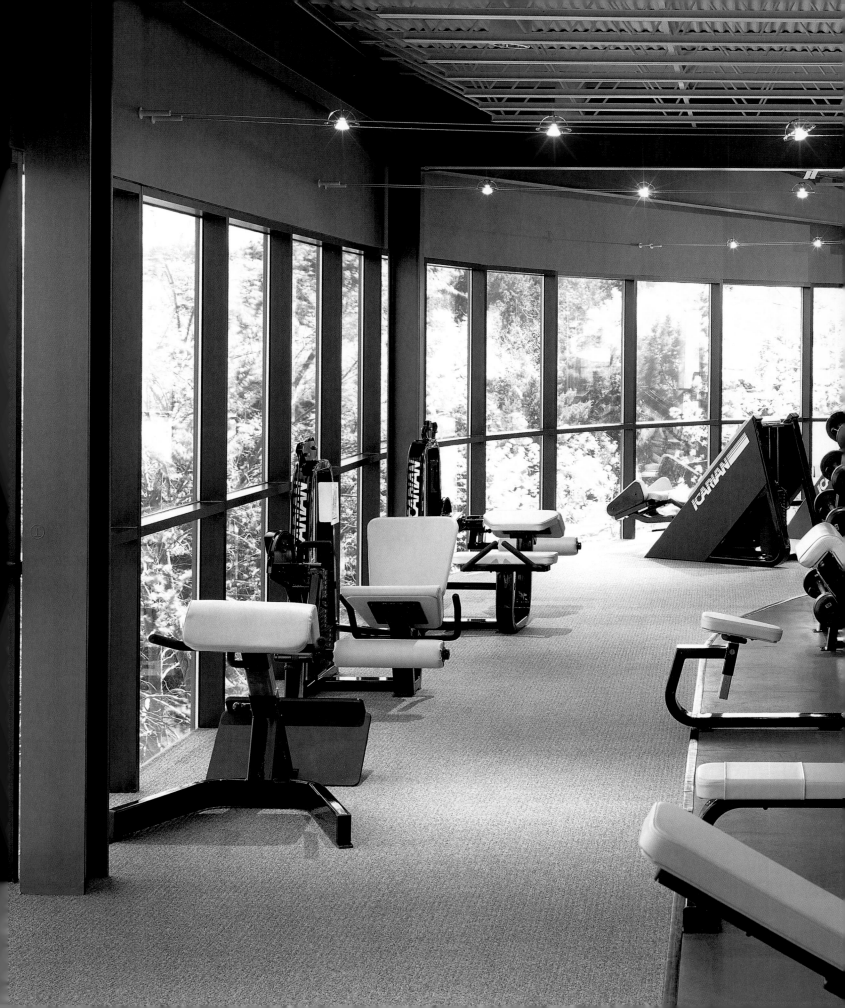

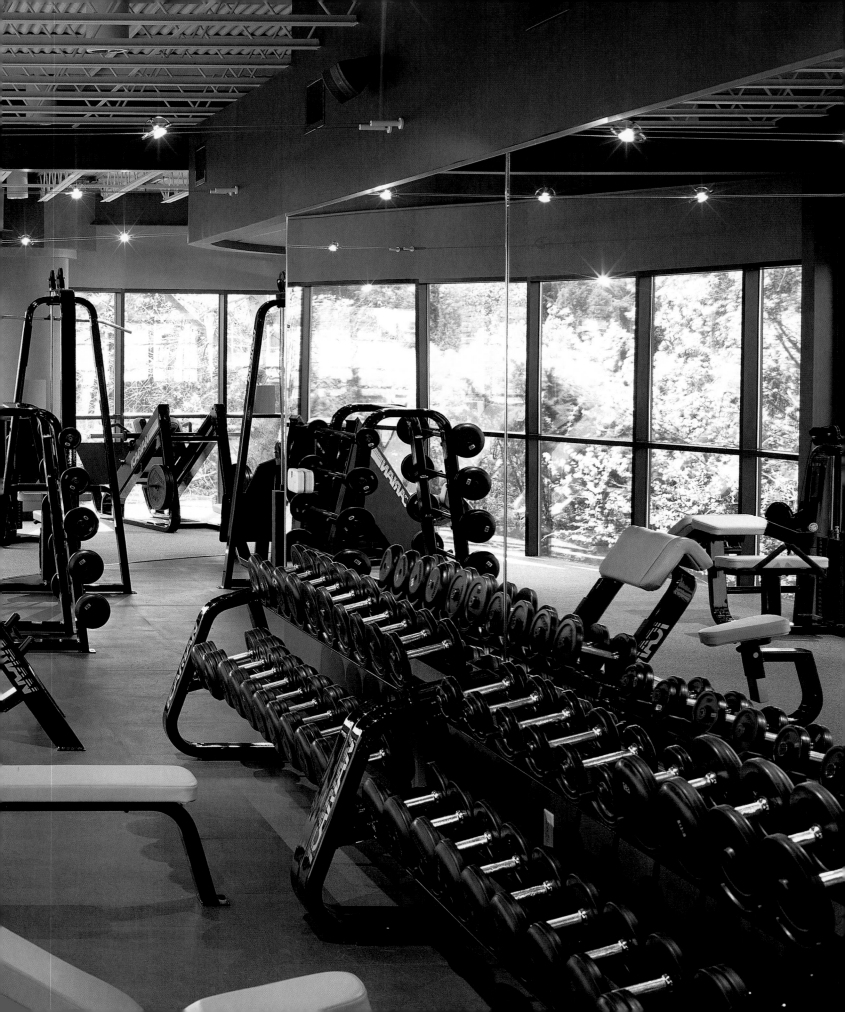

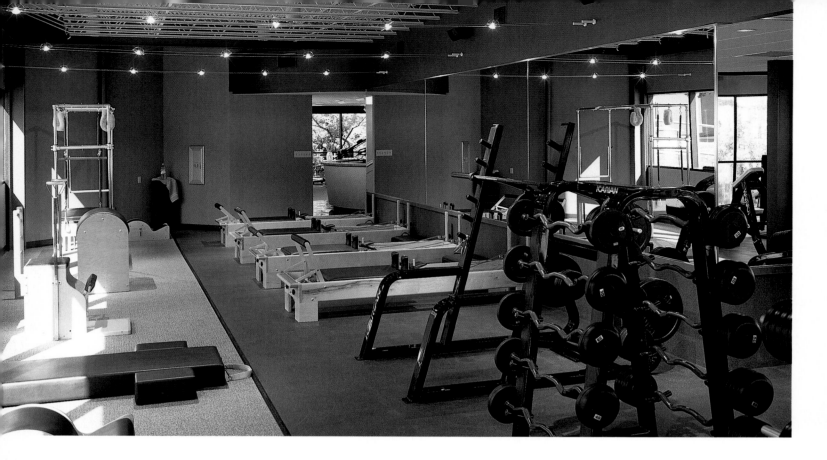

PREVIOUS SPREADS String lighting, exposed ceilings, and rubber floors create a sleek, pared-down atmosphere. The custom reception desk establishes the club's aesthetic: natural materials, clean lines, and soothing colors. Can't fight Mother Nature: wraparound windows and subtle lighting enhance the expansive views. **ABOVE** The Pilates area offers ample space for patrons and their trainers. **RIGHT** Spotless locker rooms are reduced to a few quality materials. **OPPOSITE** In the cardiovascular area, exercisers can focus on both the views and the television monitors.

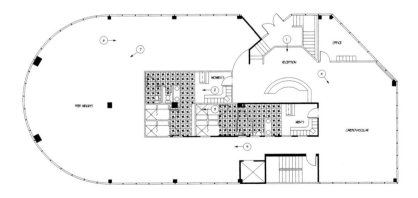

location: **Austin, Texas**
interior designer: **Peel Paulson Design Studio, Inc.**
photographer: **© 1997 Paul Bardagjy**
square feet/meters: **6,000/557**
design budget: **$1.1 million**
club membership: **250**

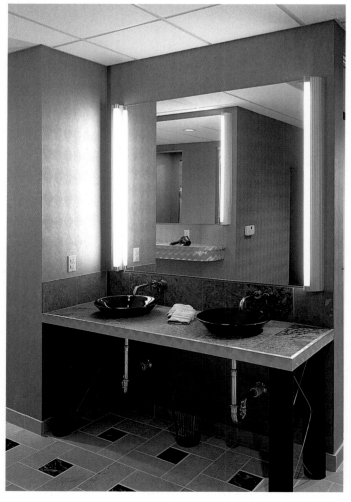

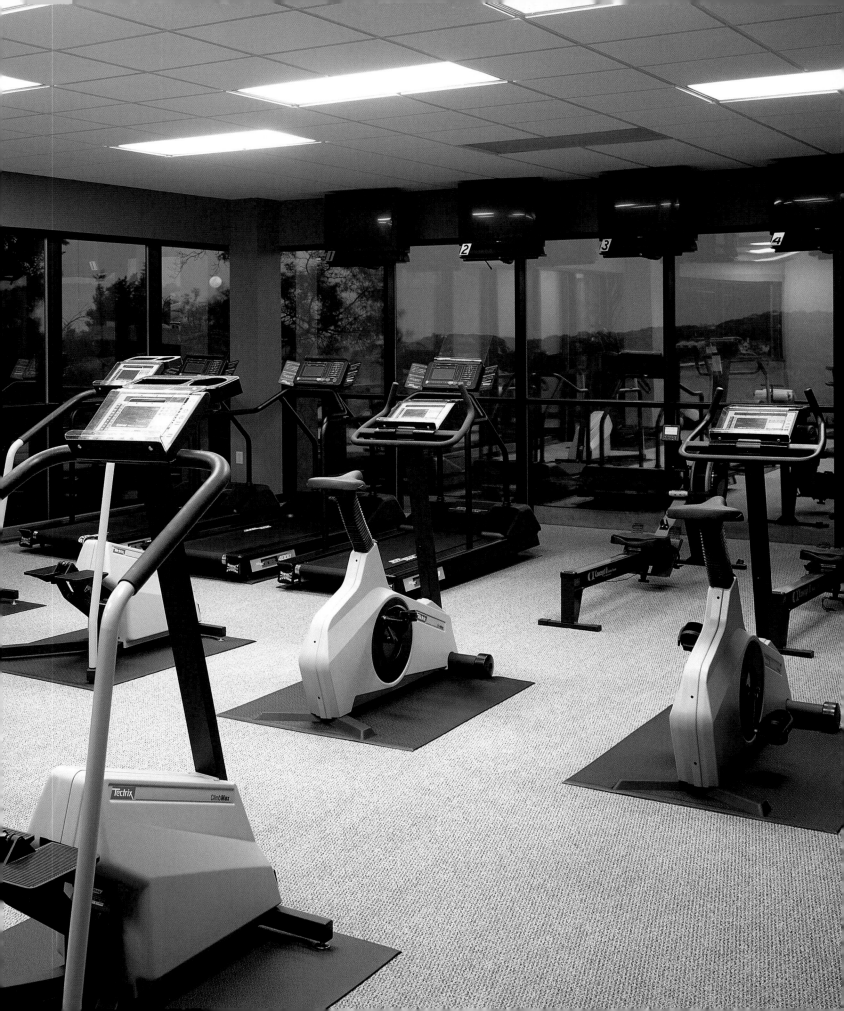

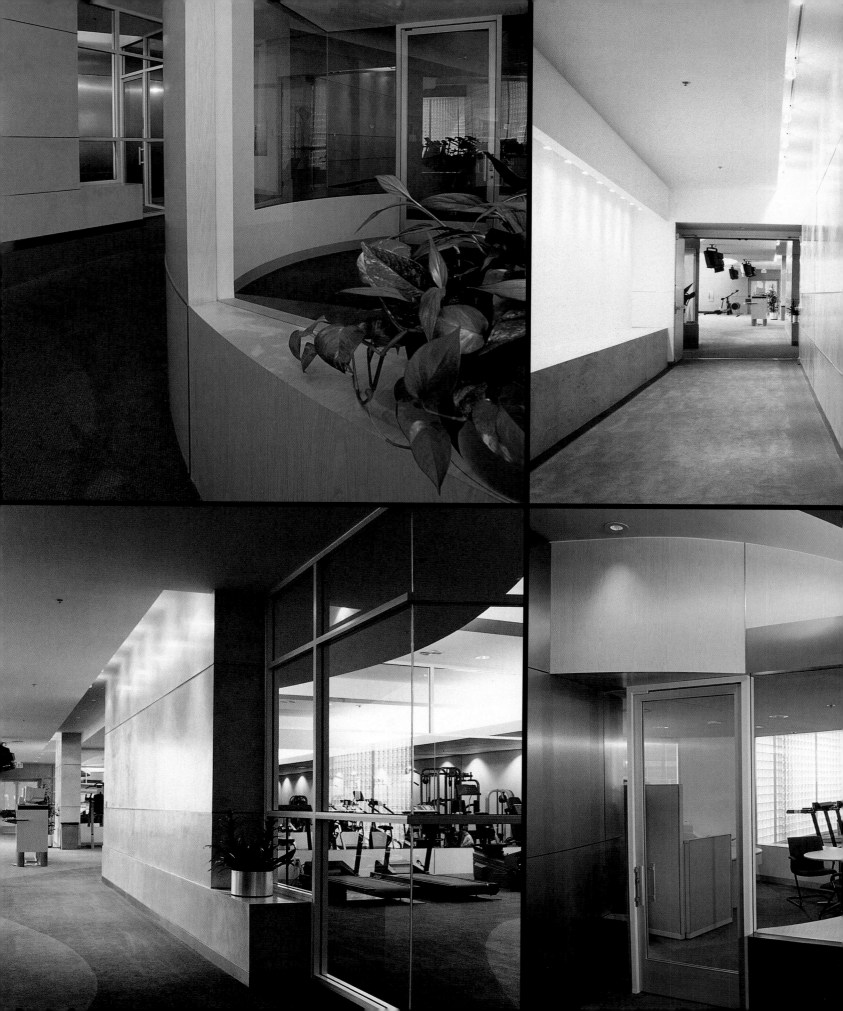

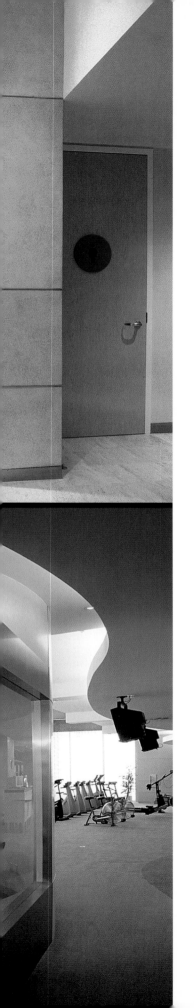

California-based toy company Mattel wanted to create a fitness center that would be a compelling gathering place for executives, creative individuals, and accountants alike. From a narrow space on the street level of a parking garage, Felderman + Keatinge Associates designed a sensuous space using rich materials, shaped by the serenity and refreshing calm of the blue sea and soft sand colors of Southern California beaches. The designers created a dialogue between hard surfaces of concrete, stainless steel, and mirrors with contrasting warm carpeting and wood tones. Though the focus is the central exercise area and examination room, curving walls prompt users to slow down and enjoy the stroll.

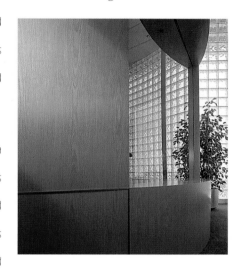

The first space one encounters is a wellness center, where employees are encouraged to research and resolve health and fitness issues through books, information, and meetings held there. Security doors lead to a corridor featuring a mural that tells the history of Mattel, created by a staff artist. Beyond the locker rooms are the examination area and exercise spaces, including weight and aerobics rooms and a separate women's gym. Careful lighting and glass block walls produce bright, welcoming interiors, while sea and beach inspire the palette. Luxe yet durable elements of stainless steel, marble, limestone, and plaster are used as accents. With a limited budget, schedule, and minimal space, Felderman + Keatinge achieved a corporate gym with surprising personality.

MATTEL HEALTH AND FITNESS CENTER

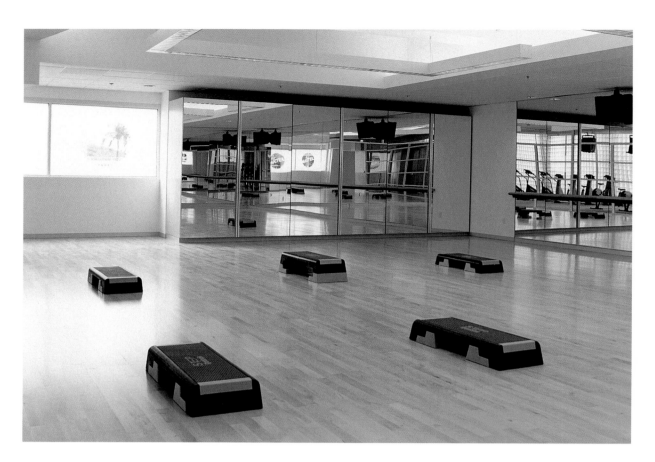

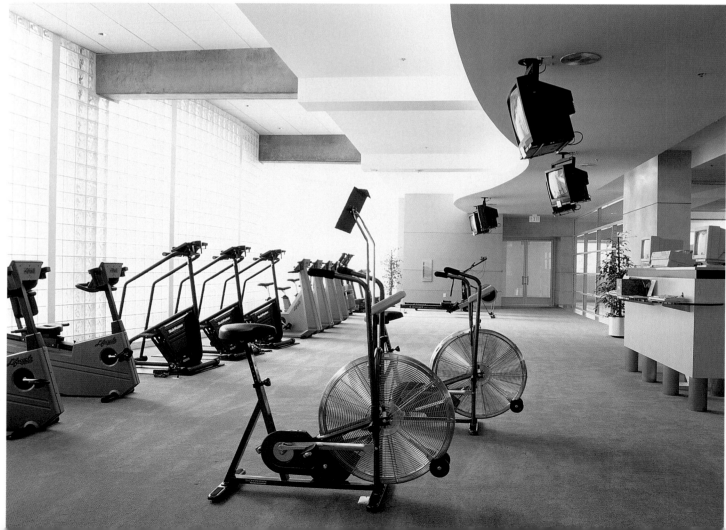

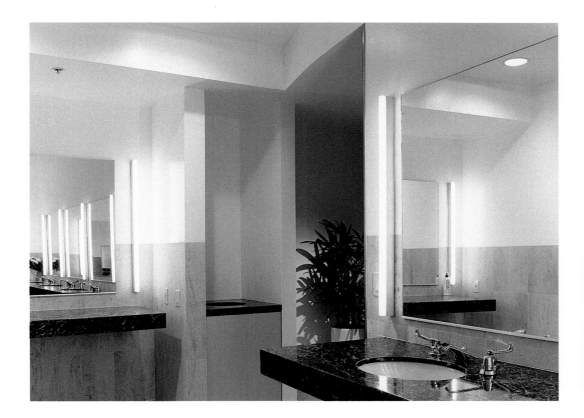
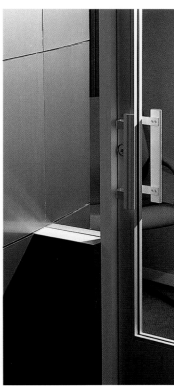

PREVIOUS SPREAD Rich yet durable elements like brushed stainless steel, pigmented plaster, and maple support the natural palette. The long, narrow gym is a progression of spaces; past the locker rooms are the women's gym and examination room, then the exercise spaces. Glass block walls and recessed lighting create bright, flattering interiors. OPPOSITE The designers created a feeling of openness to encourage staff interaction, with expansive areas and glass walls. Curved forms in the walls, ceiling, and carpet create sensuousness and invite users to relax. ABOVE Locker rooms feature opulent materials like green marble on countertops and maple cabinetry.

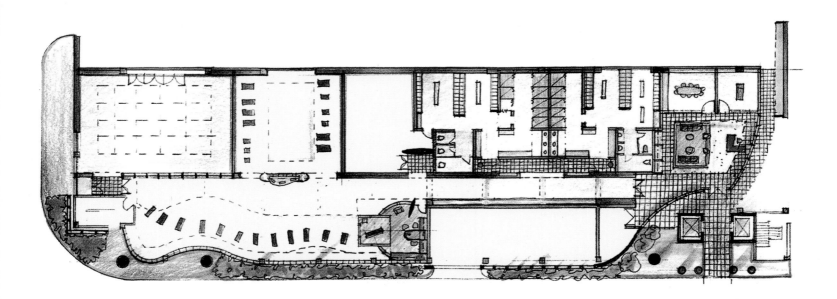

location: El Segundo, California
architect/interior designer: Felderman + Keatinge Associates
photographers: Stanley Felderman of Felderman + Keatinge Associates; Jim Sims
square feet/meters: 15,000/1,394
design budget: $1.2 million

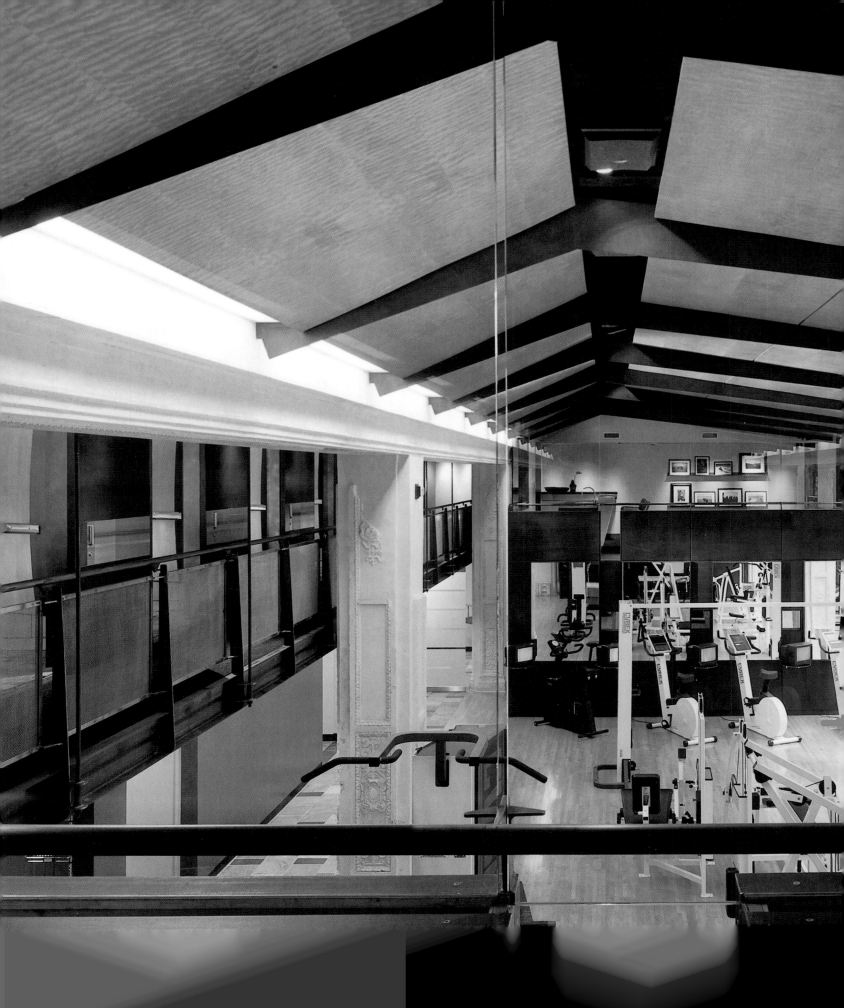

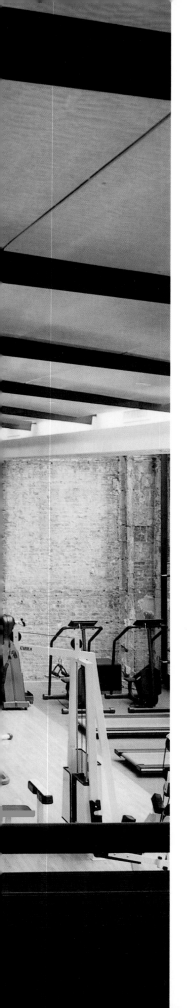

Personal trainer Pat Manocchia approached HLW International's Paul Boardman with his plans to open a revolutionary gym/clinic, dedicated to prescribed fitness as a medical pursuit. With only 300 members, La Palestra Center for Preventative Maintenance employs diagnostic and rehabilitative services, physical therapy, and a staff physiologist and cardiologist to create a program for each client. La Palestra becomes "another dimension of one's life," says Boardman.

The site was an unlikely standout—the former ballroom of the Hotel des Artistes on Manhattan's upper West Side, unrecognizable after 20 years as ABC Studios. HLW International stripped it to its essence, retaining original columns, restoring plaster walls, and uncovering a concealed 150-foot skylight. The designers created spatial tension by sliding a maple ceiling into the old shell,

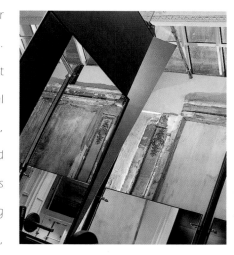

then stabilizing the shell with an artful metal framework. To provide both lofty and intimate areas, the space was bisected several times, with two large open workout areas and medical and therapy offices on the first floor. Additional offices, a library, and juice bar are located on the new mezzanine. Seven private changing rooms offer steamer trunk inspired dressers and glass showers. Materials are upscale yet functional: Indian slate tile reveals earthy tones when wet, and metal surfaces were left untreated for their cocoa hue. Custom-designed furniture adorns the lobby, juice bar, and offices.

LA PALESTRA
CENTER FOR PREVENTATIVE MAINTENANCE

location: New York, New York
architect/interior designer: HLW International LLP
photographer: © Scott Frances/Esto
square feet/meters: 15,000/1,394
design budget: $2 million
club membership: 300

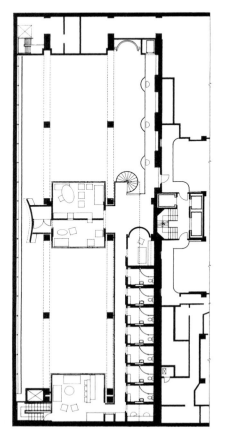

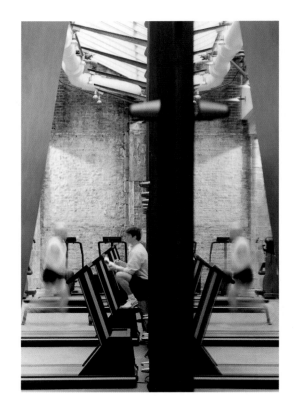

PREVIOUS SPREAD A maple ceiling was installed into the existing shell, creating tension between old and new materials. Patinated, mirrored partitions create kinetic spaces between the two main workout areas.
ABOVE The generous skylight, once concealed by the previous occupant, provides natural light in the space.
BELOW The architects added a mezzanine level where changing rooms, a library, and offices are housed.
RIGHT An original colonnade bisects the two-story space. Cardiovascular machines face mirrors hung from a new metal framework.

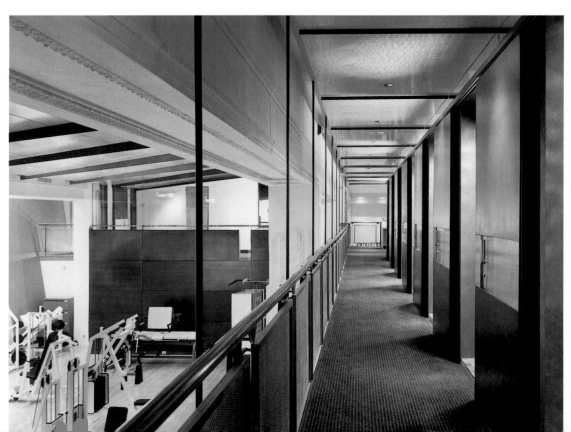

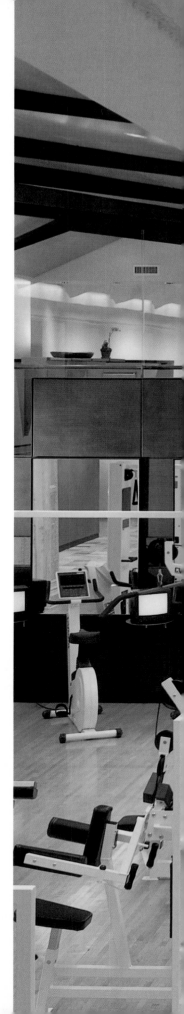

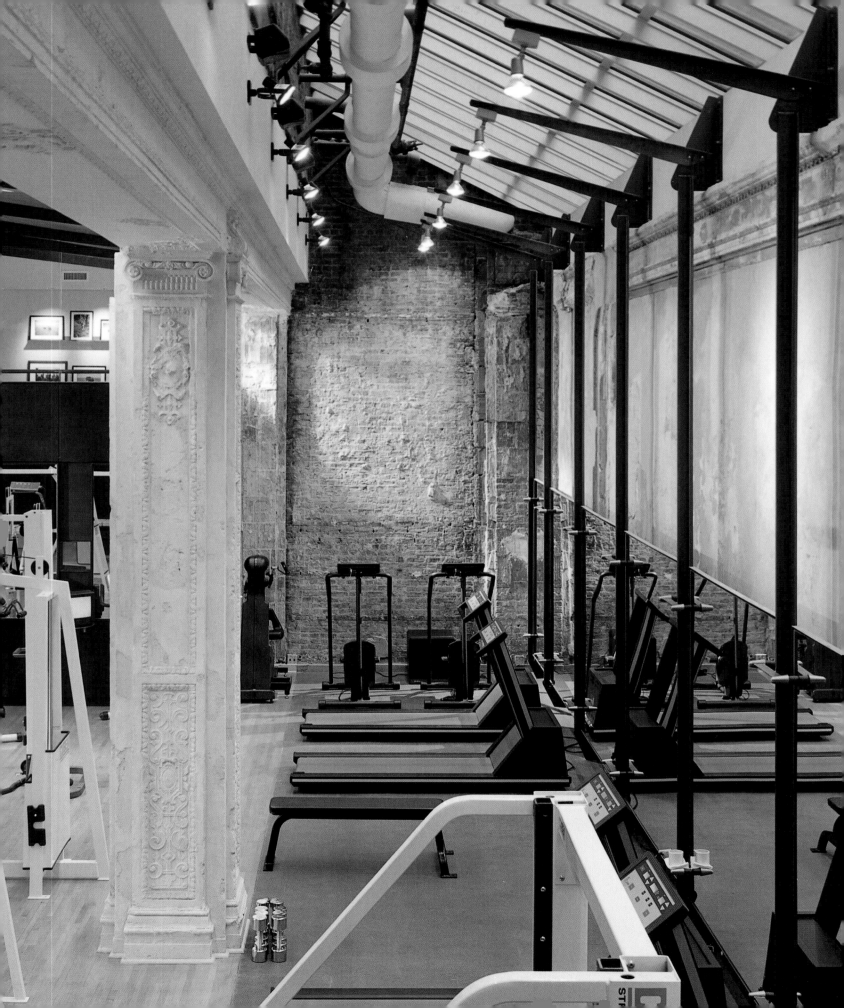

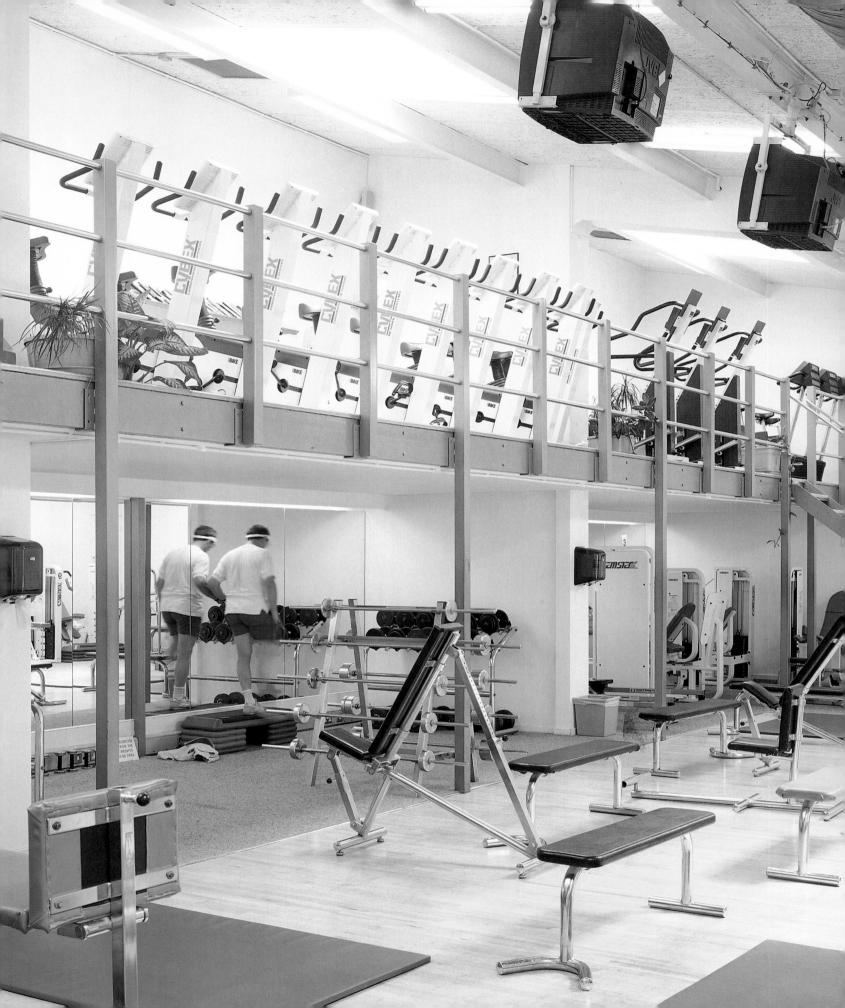

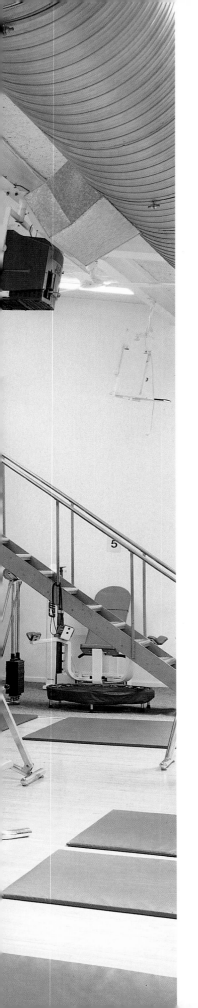

F

lexibility is the key to success for the Hogarth Group—the designers and owners of several London health clubs. The firm opened its first club, Lambton Place, in 1971 and it has evolved ever since. A good location helps: the club is in an upscale West London residential area convenient to the business community. But like many health clubs which compete for favorable sites with retail, business, and residential concerns, it has made the most of an unusual situation.

Originally constructed in 1885 as cobbled mews (garages), to house both horses and servants behind more fashionable homes, Lambton Place was purchased by a convent in 1908, and a student gymnasium was installed at the rear. When it was sold in the '60s, the poorly lit and constructed building was considered suitable for few uses—except a fitness center. The Hogarth Group reconfigured the 40-foot-high gym as a two-story squash club; later, as squash declined in popularity, the firm converted the lower courts into an

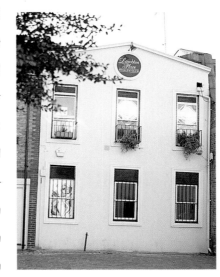

indoor pool complex and the upper courts into an open plan gym. Recently, the club added two floors. When the local council designated the neighborhood a conservation area, the Hogarth Group was required to install period-correct brickwork on the facade and slate roofing. But the interiors are modern: natural light and materials, numerous amenities, and lofty spaces attract a large base of members—even some 27-year patrons who joined when the fees were just 80 U.S. dollars a year.

LAMBTON PLACE HEALTH CLUB

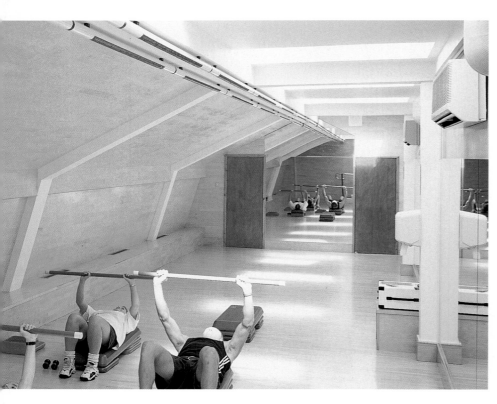

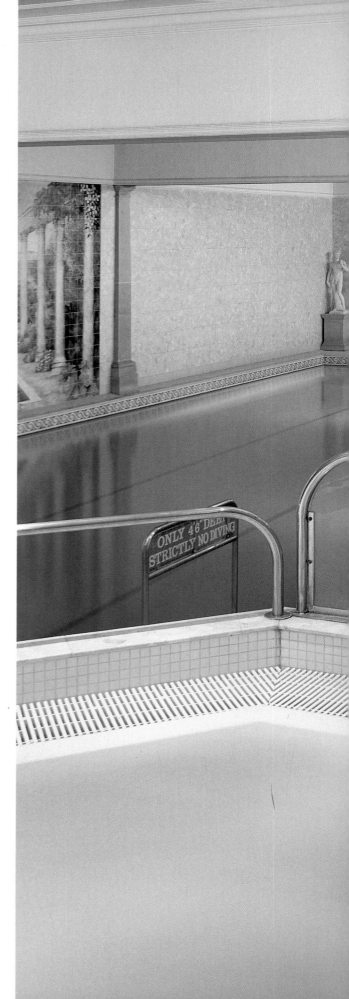

PREVIOUS SPREAD In renovating the squash courts into a gymnasium, the 18-foot-high ceilings allowed the addition of a mezzanine, which houses cardiovascular equipment. The Hogarth Group added new period-correct brickwork details and a slate roof to meet conservation laws. ABOVE Lambton Place features a sleek aerobics studio lined in maple in its new roof area. RIGHT The club offers a 60-foot indoor swimming pool, whirlpool spa, and steam room, with classical landscape murals that compensate for the lack of natural light.

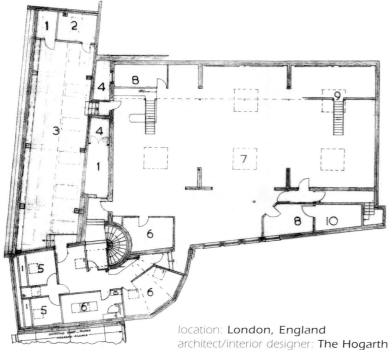

location: **London, England**
architect/interior designer: **The Hogarth Group**
photographer: **The Hogarth Group**
square feet/meters: **17,000/1600**
design budget: **$2.5 million**
club membership: **2,000**

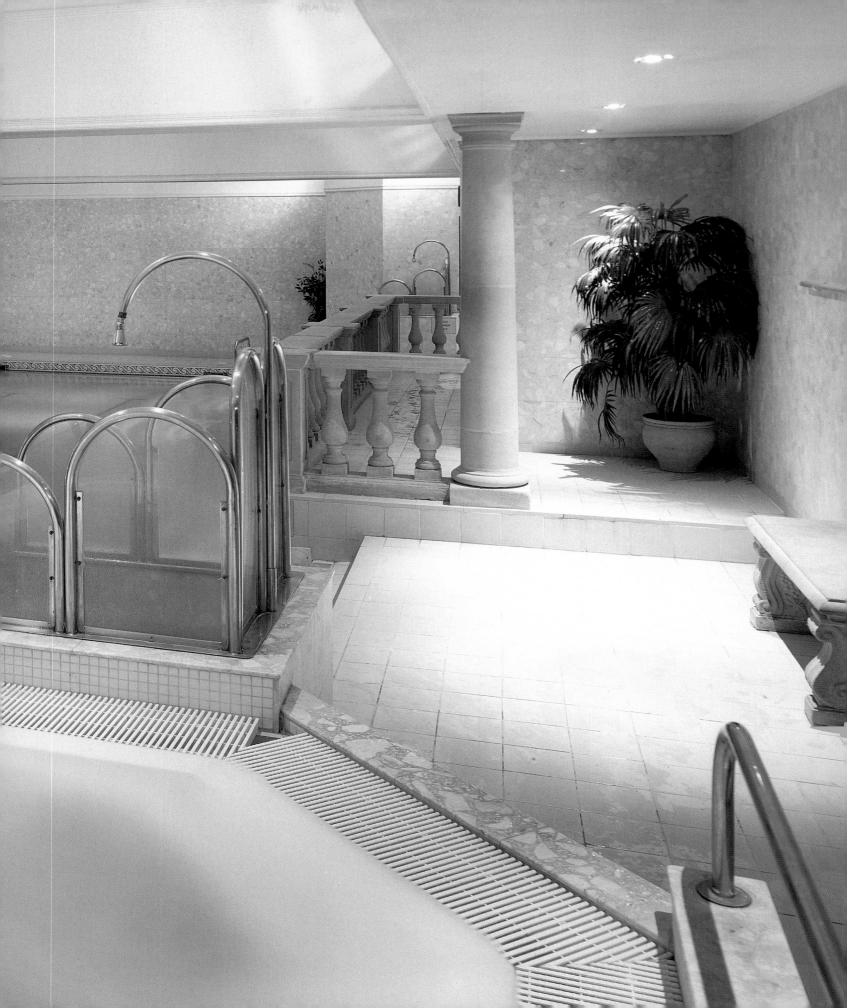

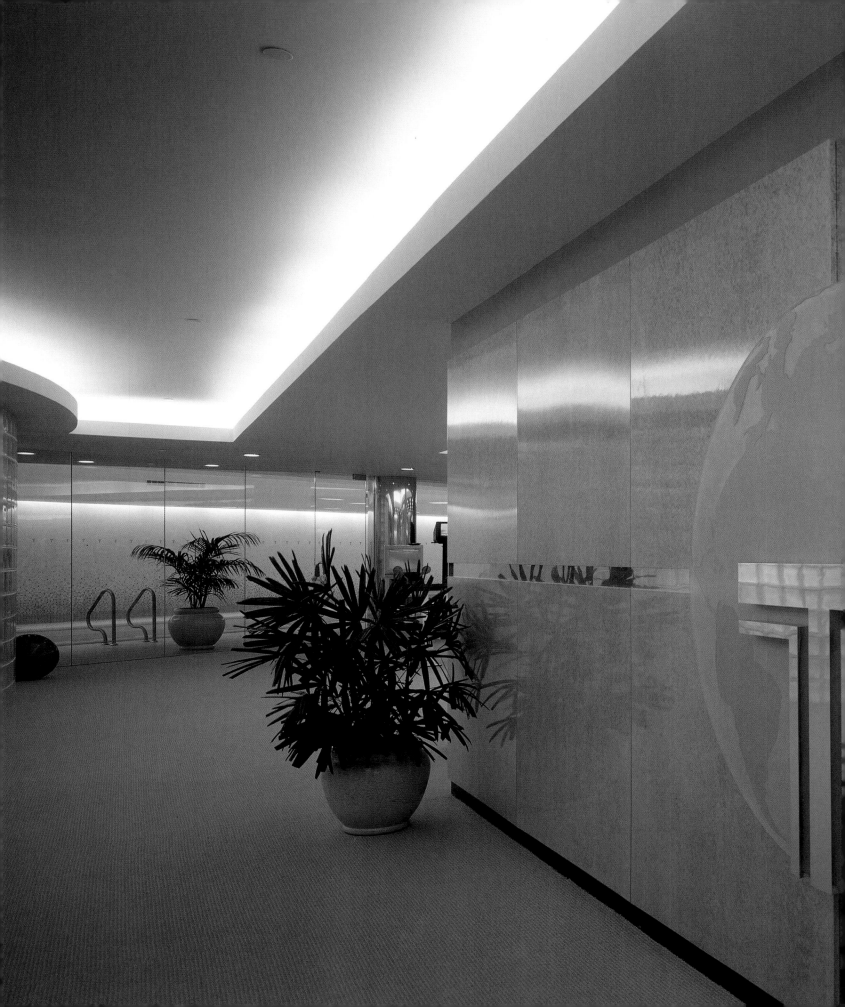

Leave it to Donald Trump to fashion a health club in his likeness: the Fitness Center and Spa at the Trump International Hotel & Tower on Central Park West sports the gold and brass detailing and subtle "T" accents that are his signature. Designers Smith-Palmer + Famulari transformed the original gym plan, which did not make the most of the cellar site, into a bright, inviting retreat for both hotel guests and residents. Principal Craig J. Smith who directed the plan, maintains that the most successful interiors are those that are "aesthetically unique yet easy to maintain."

Because the owners wanted the club to be as modern as possible, the designers focused on quality materials like anigré woods, ceramic tile, and glass block. A large yet warmly hued open area, cleared by running the cellar's piping along the perimeter and lining walls with ductwork, houses the cardiovascular and weight

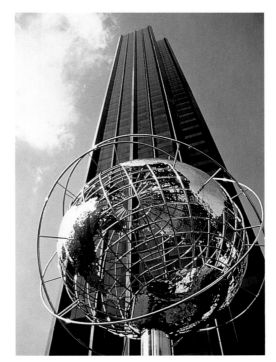

training equipment. A frameless glass wall dividing the lap pool from the workout area partitions the space. Down a curving glass block corridor are the locker rooms, featuring wood lockers with finishes of peach and burgundy, and intimate massage rooms. Indirect lighting and a sandy palette are an extension of the hotel's interiors.

TRUMP FITNESS CENTER & SPA

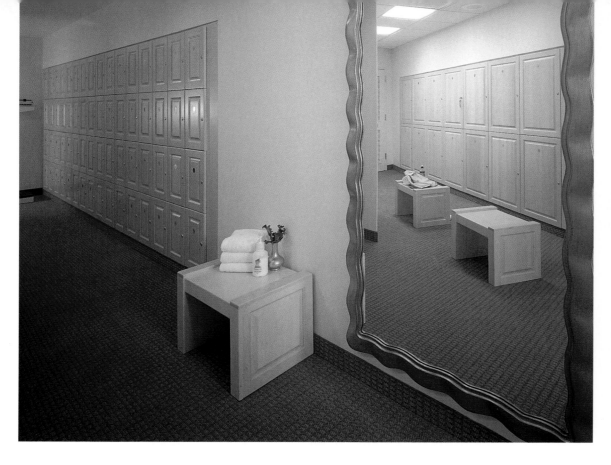

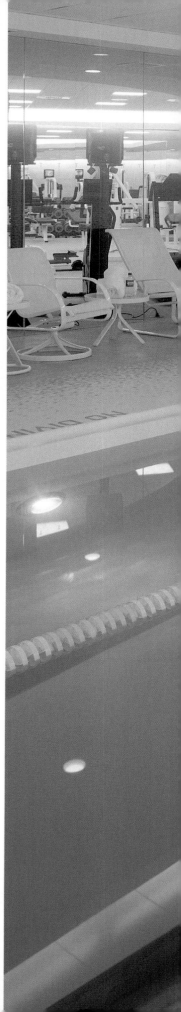

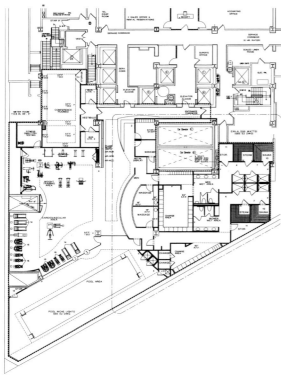

PREVIOUS SPREAD The club reception area employs natural materials, sandy tones, and signature Trump detailing. ABOVE The women's room has peach walls and wood lockers with gold-toned accents. BELOW Curving glass block walls create a dynamic passageway. RIGHT The comfortable pool area is partitioned from the cardiovascular room with a frameless glass wall.

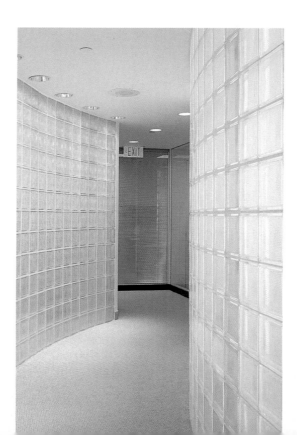

location: New York, New York
architect/interior designer: Smith-Palmer + Famulari
photographer: Philip Jensen-Carter
square feet/meters: 6,000/557
design budget: $1.8 million

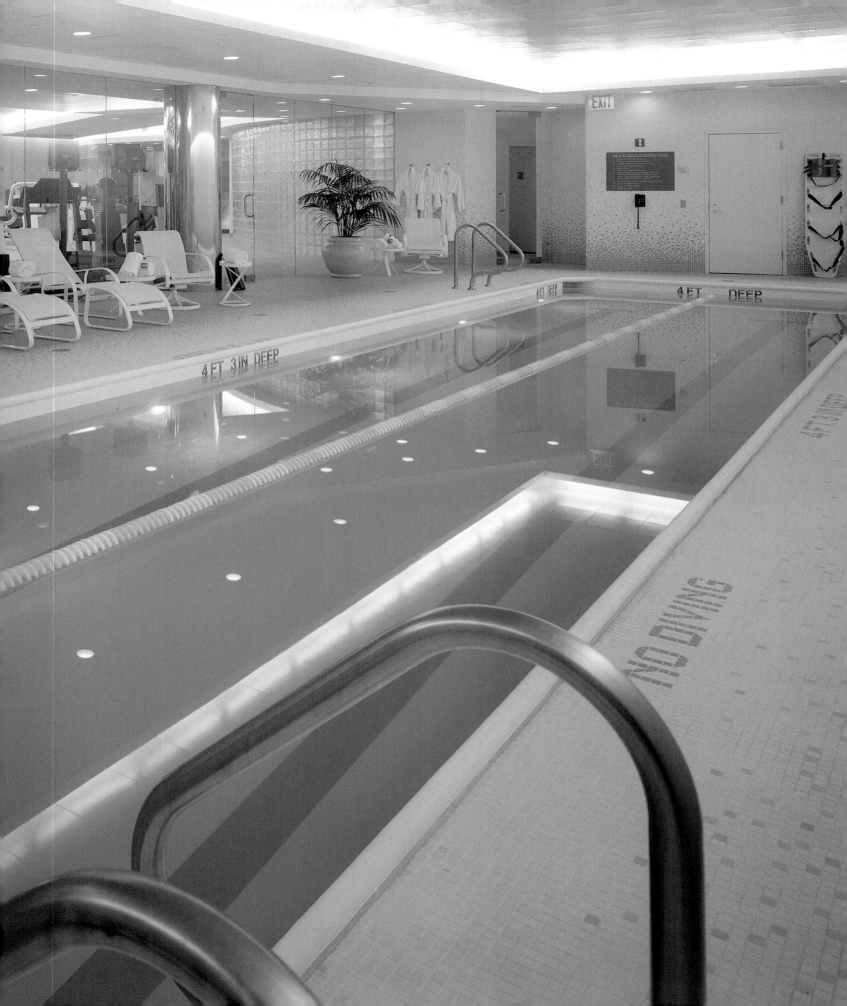

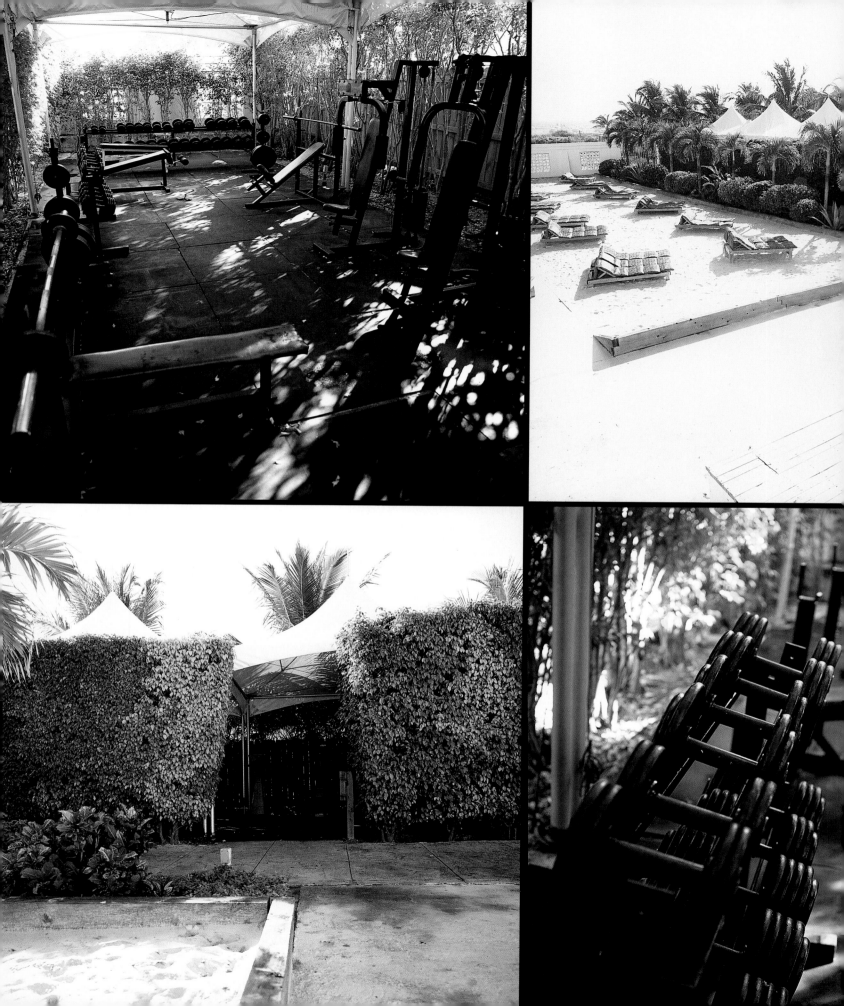

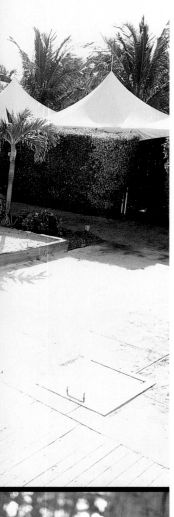

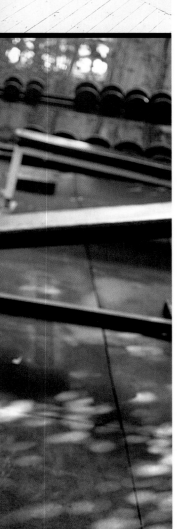

As part of the redevelopment of Miami Beach's opulent Art Deco hotels, which has once again established the district as one of America's great resort destinations, the beach-side Raleigh Hotel was recently restored to its former grandeur. Its scalloped, landscaped pool, thought by many to be the most beautiful in South Beach, was also revamped; beyond the poolside bar and sprawling lounge area lies the Atlantic Ocean.

The owner wanted to incorporate a gym within the lush grounds that would not detract from the hotel's time-honored beauty. He ingeniously created a hideaway of a gym that offers ample facilities yet embraces nature, the open air and sea breezes. The 1,500-square-foot gym is a narrow, white-tented structure, surrounded by dense full-height hedges

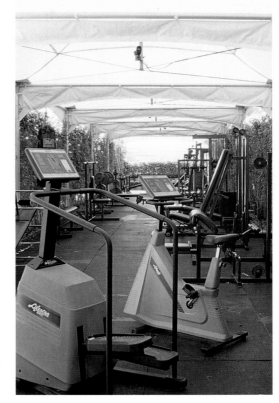

that shield from the elements and create a serene aura of dappled sunlight. Rubber flooring is employed under free weights and circuit and cardiovascular equipment to absorb shock. Guests can work out in privacy yet enjoy the outdoors, a treat for users from harsher climes.

RALEIGH FITNESS CENTER

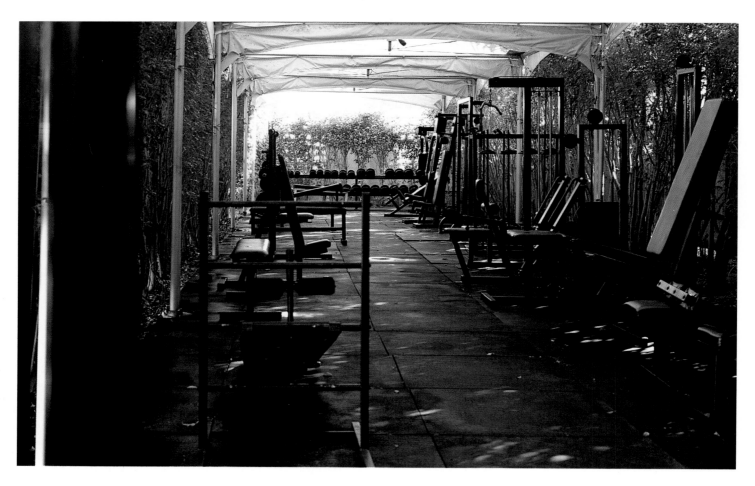

PREVIOUS SPREAD Sunlight trickles in through the hedges and from the beach side of the gym, while a tented roof and high hedge walls shield users from the elements. ABOVE Rubber flooring offers a cushion to equipment users; music is piped in through mini speakers located on the tent structure. RIGHT Cardiovascular machines are interspersed with the weight training equipment. OPPOSITE The simple yet ample gym offers both circuit and free-weight equipment.

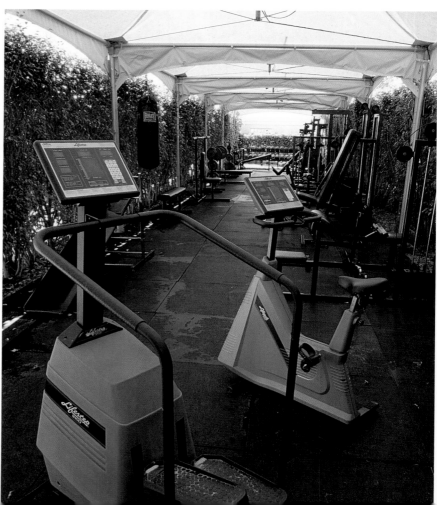

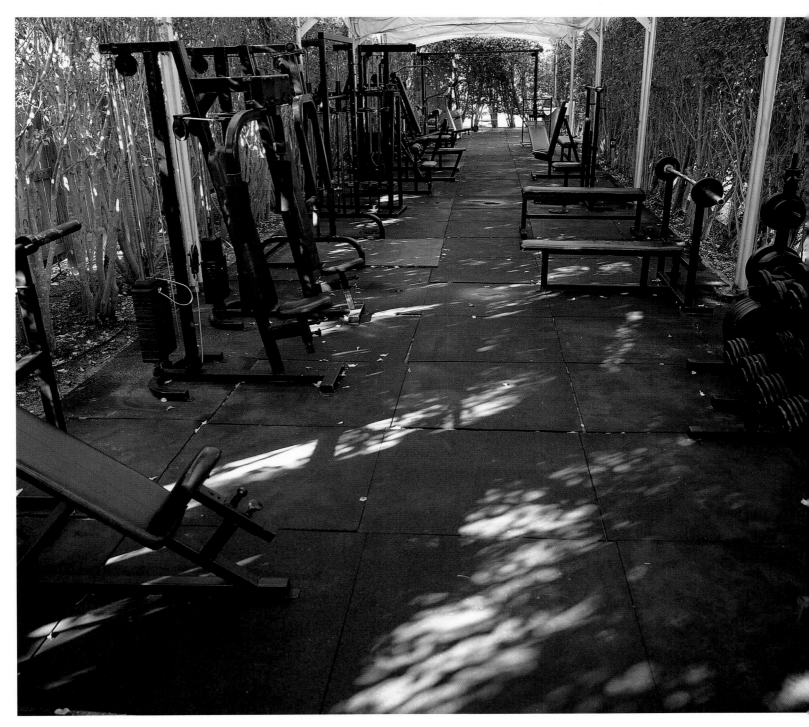

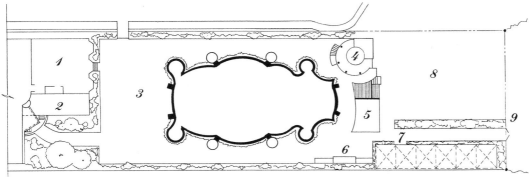

location: **Miami Beach, Florida**
interior designer: **Kenneth Zarrilli**
photographer: **A.E. Valentin**
square feet/meters: 1,500/139
design budget: $150,000
club membership: 100

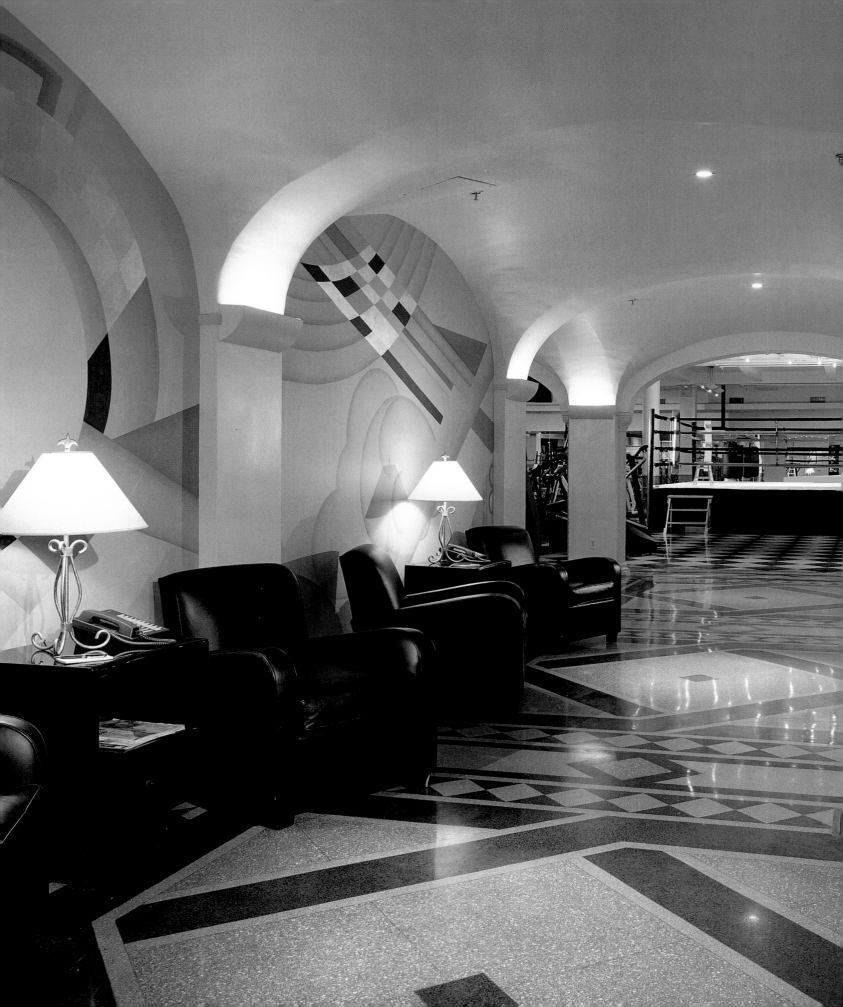

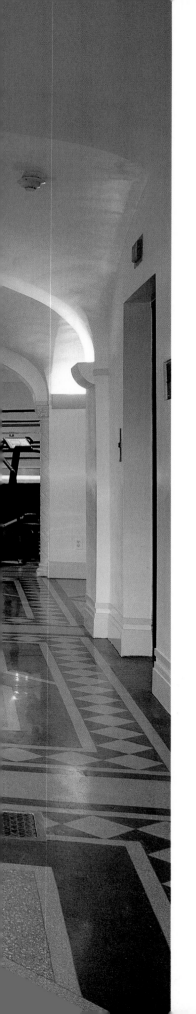

At Manhattan's Strykers Sporting Club, professional pugilists and novices alike train in atypically posh surroundings. Designed by Elevations Design & Construction, Strykers offers traditional boxing instruction with the comforts of the modern gym—perfect for health-conscious New Yorkers who also like to be pampered. In the locker rooms, clients can get a massage, hot shave, or a shoeshine. The club room offers a conference table, telephones, fax and copy machine for clients' impromptu business meetings.

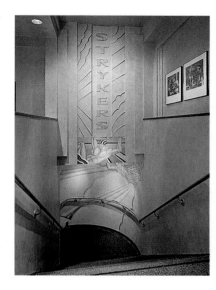

The design was largely inspired by the elements of the structure, which was occupied in the '30s and '40s by a swanky supper club. Elevations either salvaged or drew inspiration from many of the surviving Art Deco details. The reception area, created in the style of a period hotel lobby, features dramatic lighting, a sleek chrome reception desk, and a series of murals combining classical Roman images with a Machine Age aesthetic. The designers convinced the owners to restore (at great expense) the original terrazzo flooring and vaulted stucco ceilings, which cued the color palette.

The main workout floor features a large boxing area, with a regulation-size ring and several types of punching bags. The glass-walled club room overlooks the workout floor where vintage boxing posters and memorabilia collected by the designers are displayed. The locker rooms combine sensuous materials such as limestone, chrome, and velvet for durable luxury.

STRYKERS SPORTING CLUB

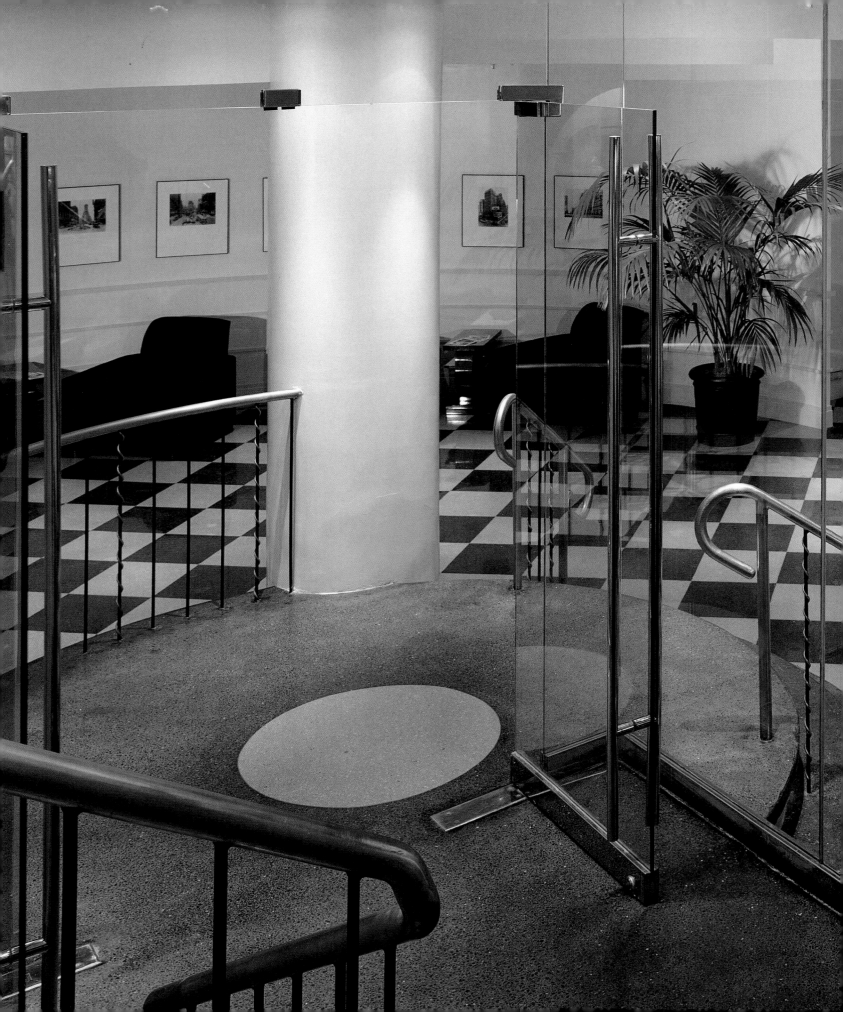

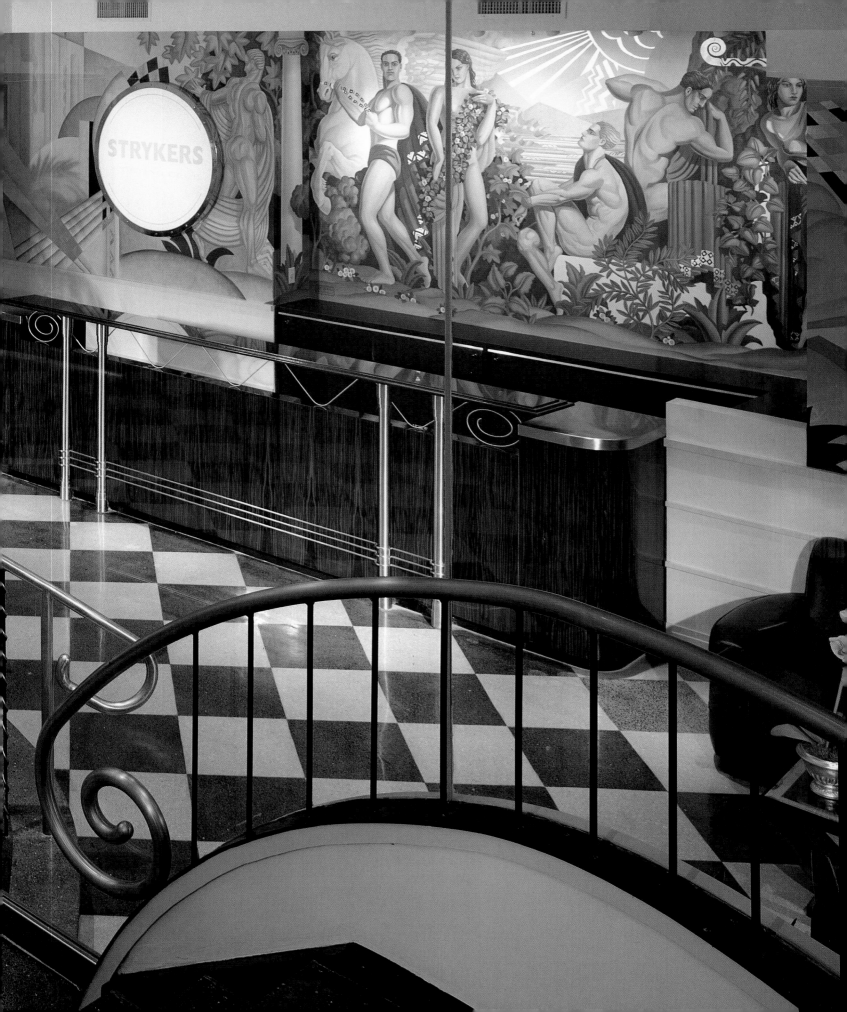

location: **New York, New York**
interior designer: **Elevations Design & Construction Co.**
photographer: **Peter Paige**
square feet/meters: **11,000/1,022**
design budget: **$3 million**
club membership: **3,000**

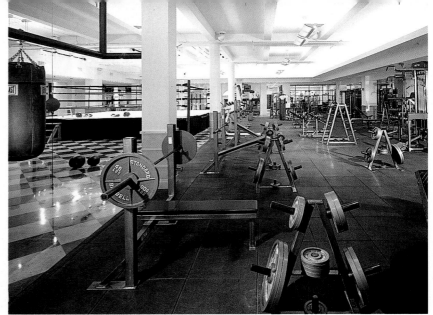

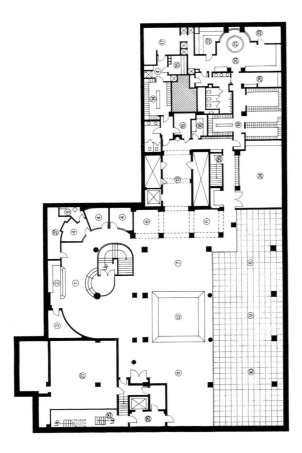

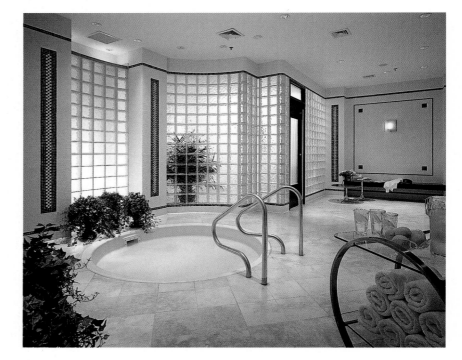

PREVIOUS SPREADS *The elevator lobby offers a quiet retreat, with leather chairs and telephones. The reception area's centerpiece is a series of murals that celebrate the human body.* **ABOVE RIGHT & OPPOSITE** *The main workout floor can be transformed into a five hundred-seat arena for sparring and boxing matches.* **CENTER RIGHT** *A glass-tiled whirlpool and steam room soothes tired bodies.* **RIGHT** *Luxe details and sensuous materials create an alluring women's locker room.*

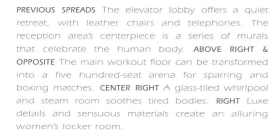

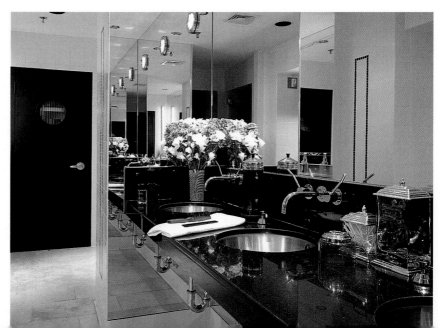

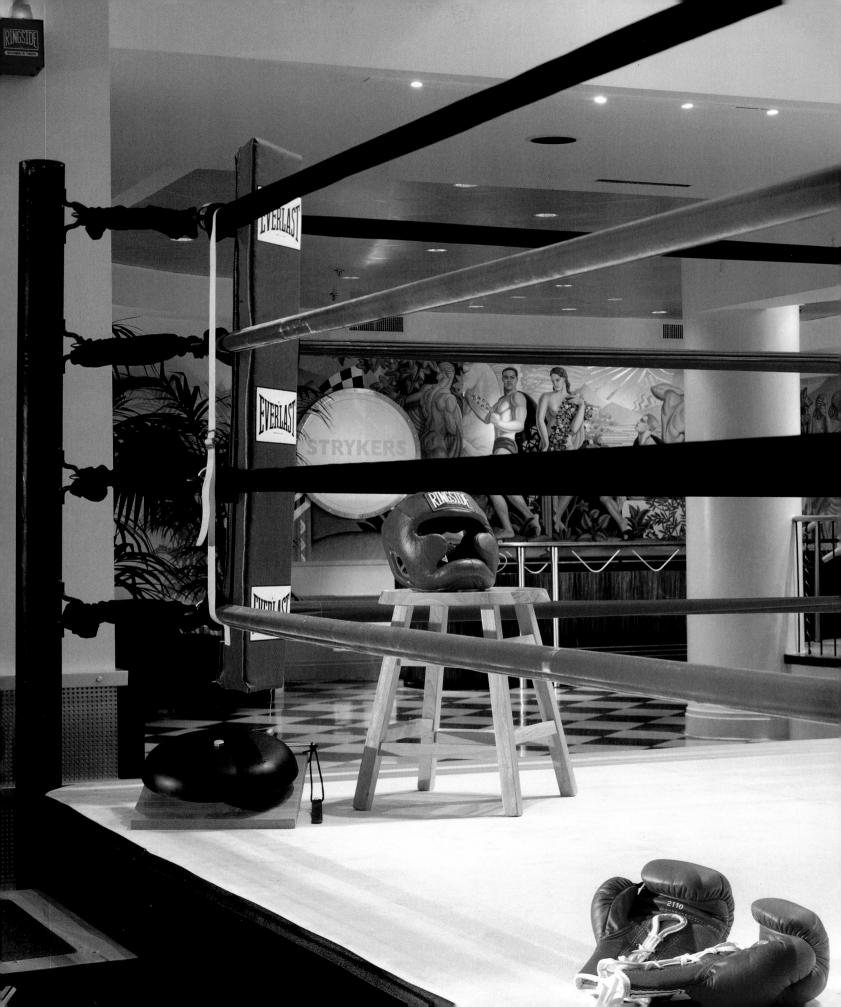

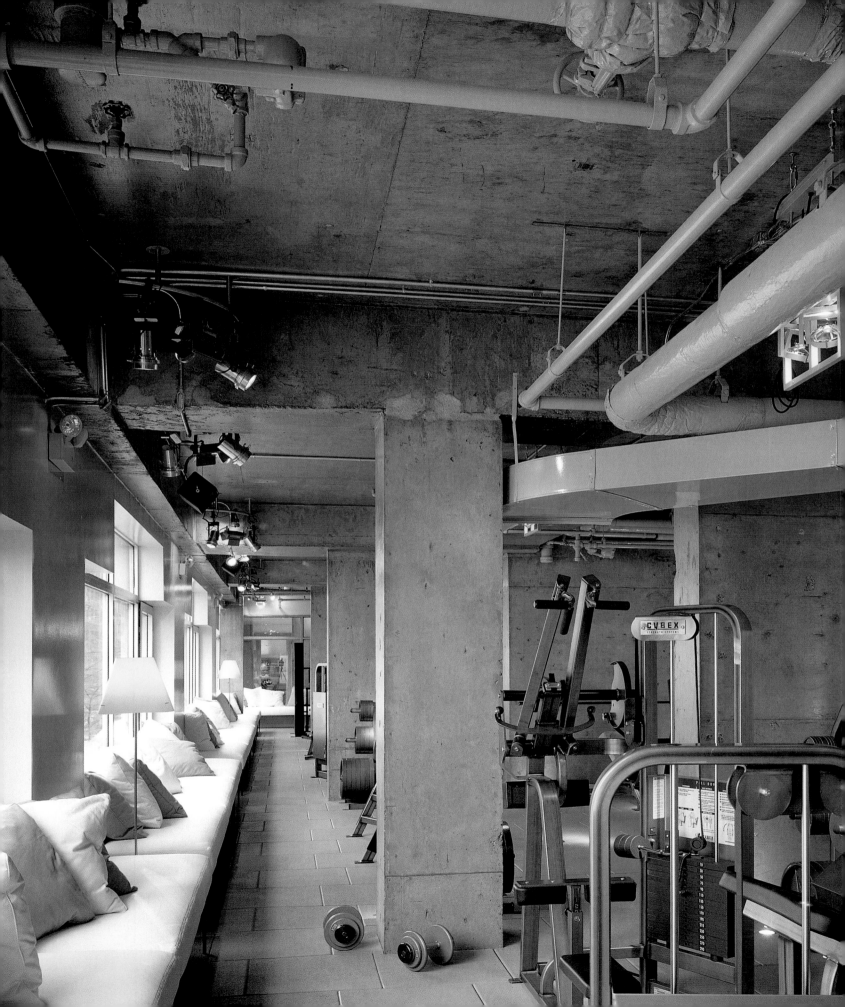

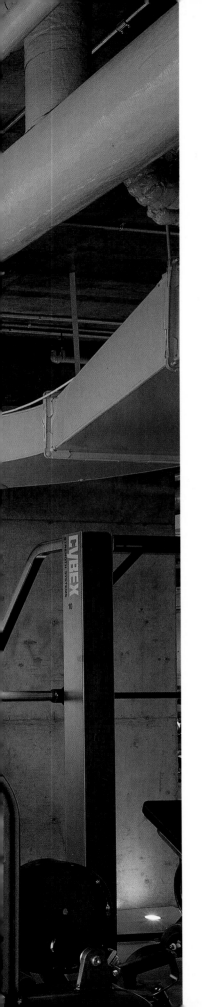

D avid Barton, charismatic owner of one of Manhattan's coolest downtown gyms, wanted to open an upper East Side location, but knew his edgy nightclub aesthetic would need rethinking. Barton approached Aero Studios, the SoHo firm known for their sophisticated residences and retail projects, to design their first gym; out of raw concrete emerged an elegant, womb-like space with layers of detail and luxurious materials.

Natural elements and other formerly taboo touches abound: the street-level entrance features a Lucite and iron desk, antique lamps, a leather banquette, industrial fans, and fir flooring, spotlighting Aero's brand of style and function. The second floor was subdivided into human-scaled areas for reception, cardiovascular, weight training,

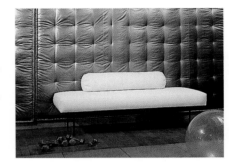

and aerobics studios, with the weight areas cached into intimate rooms. Wrapping the perimeter are a window wall and cushioned banquette where clients can lounge or socialize.

To complement the lacquered steel gym equipment and rubber floors, the white walls turn a deeper gray as one penetrates the space. Silvery tufted vinyl wall pads and metallic vinyl coverings layered throughout the gym are soft yet sleek. A residential atmosphere replaces mirrored walls in the weight areas, with wood framed mirrors and a large silver-leaf painting. In the locker rooms, Aero expressed Barton's yen for transparency by separating the men's and women's showers with a five-layer translucent glass laminate. Lighting by Johnson Schwinghammer eases from natural light to nocturnal glow.

DAVID BARTON GYM

PREVIOUS SPREAD Residential touches contrast with rubber flooring, exposed concrete walls, and pipes. RIGHT Barton's office features wood casing and vintage furniture, two elements formerly taboo in health clubs. BELOW The street-level entrance has a custom Lucite and iron desk instead of a standard monolithic check-in desk. OPPOSITE ABOVE The weight-training areas feature randomly placed wood framed mirrors, and a mesmerizing gesso and silver-leaf painting by artist Nancy Lorenz. OPPOSITE BELOW LEFT Filtered lighting is adjustable by varying colored gels. OPPOSITE BELOW RIGHT The men's shower area features an illuminated frosted glass and aluminum ceiling, and randomly placed mirror tiles pepper the walls.

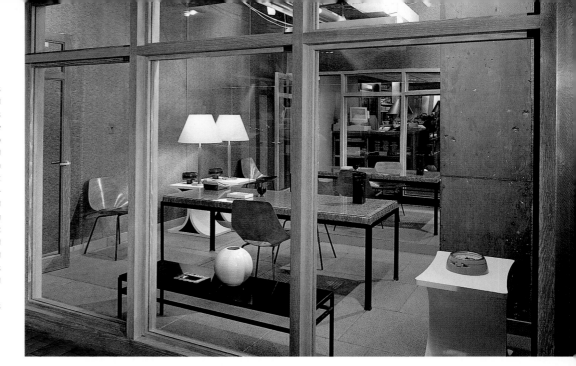

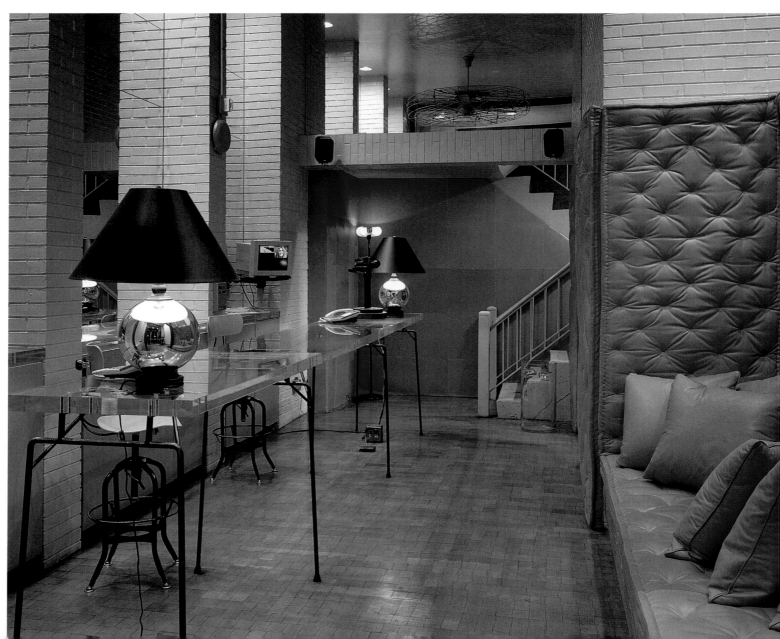

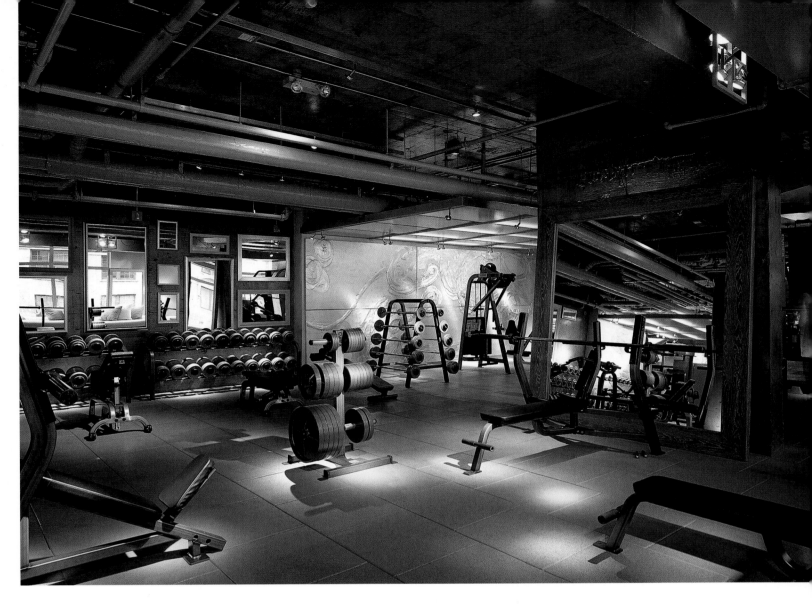

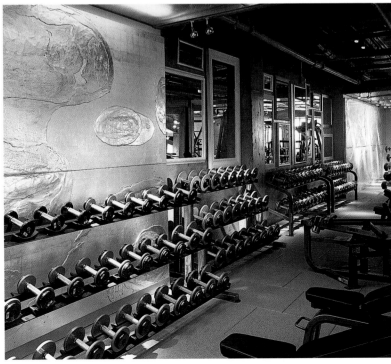

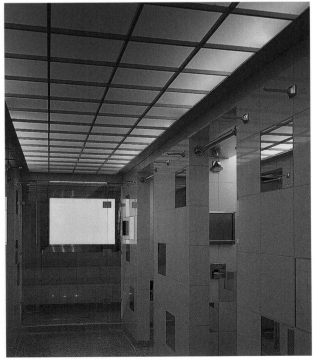

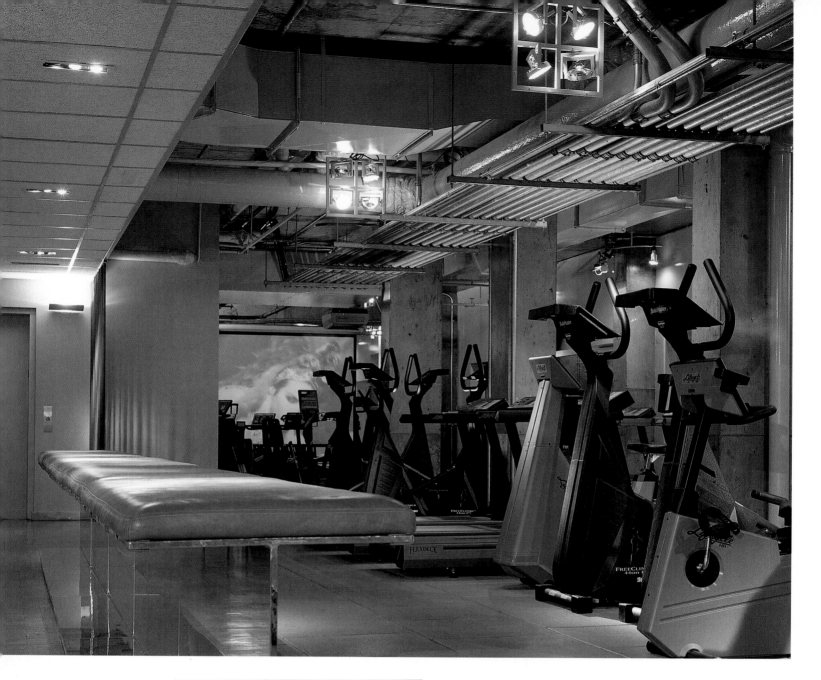

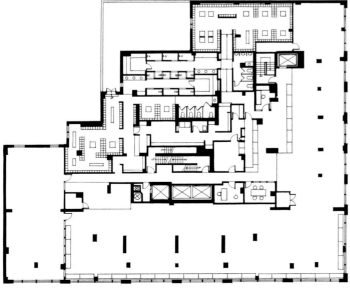

ABOVE A custom leather cushion and aluminum I-beam bench divide the cardiovascular area from reception; at rear, an oversized screen shows television and video. RIGHT In the locker rooms, Aero installed custom chrome-plated lockers to add metallic richness. Wood floors are a warm, natural element.

location: **New York, New York**
architect/interior designer: **Aero Studios Limited**
photographer: © Peter Mauss/Esto
square feet/meters: 12,400/1,152
design budget: $2.5 million
club membership: 2,300

HEALTH CLUBS

ARCHITECTS AND INTERIOR DESIGNERS

PHOTOGRAPHERS

ACKNOWLEDGMENTS

My sincere thanks to the architects and interior designers whose incredible work inspired this book. My appreciation also to the talented photographers; wordless, the book would be complete.

Thank you also to the staff at PBC International, whose belief in the idea strengthened mine. And to the staff at *Interiors* magazine, especially M J Madigan and Chris Howland, whose advice—and flexibility—made the project possible.

And last to my husband, who gladly shared the planning of our wedding with the writing of a book, and who cheers me on in every race.

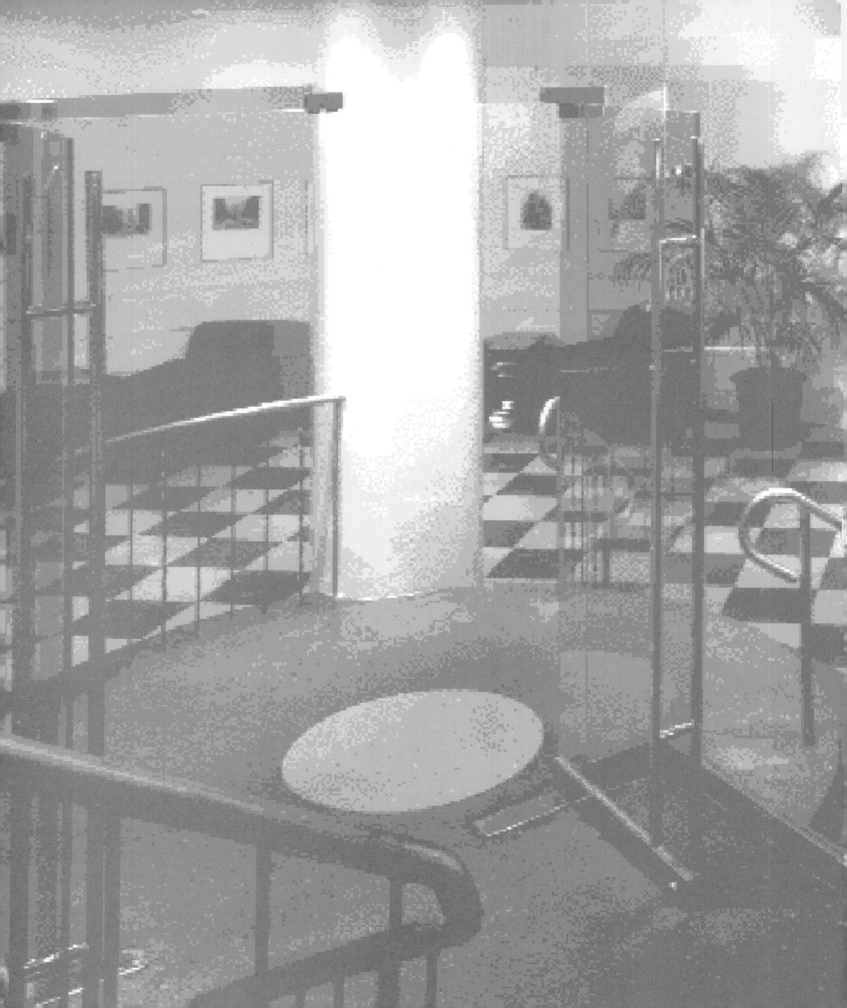